THE VITAMIN REVOLUTION
IN HEALTH CARE

by

MICHAEL JANSON, M.D.

ARCADIA PRESS
Greenville, New Hampshire

Cover design: Foster and Foster, Inc., Fairfield, Iowa
Cover photo: Koby-Antupit Photographers

Publisher's Cataloging-in-Publication Data

Janson, Michael, 1944-
    The vitamin revolution in health care / Michael Janson.
    p. cm.
    Includes bibliographical references and index.
    ISBN 0-9649236-9-6 (Paperback)
    ISBN 0-9649236-8-8 (Hardbound)

    1. Dietary supplements. 2. Vitamins. 3. Vitamin therapy.
    I. Title
    RA784.J36 1996   615.8'54
                                 QBI95-20580

Library of Congress Catalog Card Number   95-81032
                                            CIP

    97 98 99   10 9 8 7 6 5 4

Printed in the United States of America.

Ordering information:

Single copies and quantity discounts are available from the publisher, Arcadia Press, PO Box 205, Greenville, NH 03048. Telephone: 800-398-8851 or 603-878-1561.

Linus Pauling, PhD
1901-1994

To Linus Pauling, whose warmth, humanity, intellect, humor, caring, and perseverence inspired me and several generations of professionals in the biological and physical sciences. His positive influence will be felt by many generations to come.

Acknowledgements

It is impossible to list all the people who have contributed to the many years of development of this book. First is Kaare Bolgen who started me on this path. Equally important are all of my colleagues in the field of nutrition and preventive medicine, especially Michael Schachter, MD, Warren Levin, MD, and Jeffrey Bland, PhD, all of whom contributed to my education in various ways. Elmer Cranton, MD, and Jim Frackelton, MD, furthered my understanding of free radicals in health and disease.

The American College for Advancement in Medicine provided me a professional "home" for what seemed radical ideas in the past but are now becoming increasingly accepted in the medical profession. What I learned by lecturing to ACAM doctors has helped shape this book. My many patients provided me with the clinical evidence of the value of dietary supplements in medicine.

I thank Barbara Cohen and Susan Rohrbach for their thorough manuscript reviews and constructive comments, and my editor, Janis Walworth who helped clarify the difficult parts of the manuscript and picked up all those little details. Thanks to the family of the late Linus Pauling for permission to reprint Dr. Pauling's letter.

Last and perhaps most important to the completion of the book, warmest thanks to my publisher, Varuni Roberts, of Arcadia Press, without whom I never would have affixed myself to my chair to finish the writing.

Michael Janson, MD

Contents

Chapter 9 113
Flavonoids, Herbs and Botanicals

Chapter 10 133
Practical Guidelines: Buying and Taking Supplements

Foreword

Michael Janson is my friend and colleague, and we belong to a small but growing fraternity of physicians. Of the 530,000 practicing physicians in this country, Dr. Janson and I are a part of a group of perhaps only one percent—several thousand doctors—who believe that nutrition and appropriate use of vitamins, minerals and medicinal herbs should be the primary therapy for almost all of the medical conditions presented to us by our patients. This does not mean that we do not use prescription drugs, only that they are not our primary therapy .

Most of the physicians in this fraternity have the following characteristics:

1. We use very similar approaches. Almost all of us routinely prescribe esoteric dietary supplements, such as coenzyme Q10, L-carnitine, taurine, arginine, pygeum and hawthorne, in addition to more common nutrients. We often use intravenous vitamins and minerals and EDTA chelation therapy for vascular disease.

2. We come from all disciplines in medicine. Dr. Janson studied pathology, I had training in orthopedic surgery, and our ranks include psychiatrists, internists, family practitioners, and surgical sub-specialists of all varieties.

3. As a rule, we have very little, if any, hospital practice or affiliation. In general, the nature of our practices, emphasizing nutrition as primary therapy, often renders a hospital a hostile environment.

4. As Dr. Janson so clearly states, we not only do what we preach, but preach what we do. The reason for this is quite simple. Those of us with this inclination in our medical practices want exactly what our patients want, and that is optimum health with a vibrant lifestyle.

5. However, the single most consistent similarity of the handful of us who are using nutrition and dietary supplements as our primary therapy is that, like moths to the flame, we are attracted to what works.

The nutritional therapies that we use and that Dr. Janson writes about in this book have a strong, in fact, irrefutable basis in science and the medical literature. That they are ignored by the overwhelming majority of conventional physicians is testimony to the power of the institutionalized bias instilled by a medical education system that is virtually controlled by the large pharmaceutical companies.

In addition, for a doctor to structure a practice around the tenets of nutrition puts him or her at professional risk of censure by the state agencies that control the medical profession. As Benjamin Rush, a physician and signer of the Declaration of Independence, once said, "Unless we put medical protection into the Constitution, the time will come when medicine will organize into an undercover dictatorship." This has, without question, occurred, and the forces of the American Medical Association, the Food and Drug Administration (FDA) and the pharmaceutical industry often create awesome hurdles for physicians like us to overcome.

Challenges to medical dogma of any era always meet resistance, but never at any time in history has so much money been at stake. As Dr. Janson clearly points out in this book, nutrition and nutritional supplements can be used for the very conditions that are currently being treated with large amounts of prescription drugs, and it is a decidedly uneven playing field.

The financial power of the drug manufacturers literally dwarfs the entire nutritional supplement industry. Most large drug companies have a single pharmaceutical, whether it's Tagamet®, Zantac®, Prozac®, or Cardizem®, which by itself garners gross sales above $5-$10 billion. *The entire nutritional supplement industry is only $4.6 billion.* Yet Dr. Janson convincingly argues, that various nutritional supplements can be used as treatment of the same conditions that are currently being treated with drugs, and that the nutritional approach is more successful, less expensive and infinitely safer.

These forces are evident in Dr. Janson's writings. For years, Dr. Janson has argued the obvious to those mired in the old dogma, and he is doing it again in his book because he knows that we are slowly but surely gaining ground.

Dr. Janson clearly presents the need for nutritional supplementation. It is now a superstition to think that one can get all the nutrients for optimum health from diet alone. The quality of our diet is deteriorating rapidly, and the toxicity of our environment is constantly increasing. In addition, true preventive medicine is not a string of negatives, such as "don't eat fat," "don't smoke," and "don't abuse alcohol." It is more a pro-active lifestyle, with exercise, diet, and nutritional supplementation being used in the never-ending, yet fruitful quest for optimum health.

Dr. Janson quickly lays to rest the common fallacy that those who take vitamins do so in order to excuse or overcome a poor diet. Exactly the opposite is usually the case: those who take supplements are also most likely to eat whole, nutritious foods. Dr. Janson also points out the silliness of the Recommended Dietary Allowances (RDA), which are arbitrarily kept low in order to make processed food appear healthier than it actually is. In short, Dr. Janson's book is a treatise of specific recommendations on how to use nutritional supplements to nurture your system and achieve optimum health.

The Vitamin Revolution is extremely well organized and easy to read. There is obvious and expected repetition among different dietary supplement programs for specific problems because a host of degenerative diseases result from similar nutritional weaknesses. The book is valuable for both the general public and the physician.

Finally, Dr. Janson clearly points out the political repression of the nutritional supplement industry by the FDA. In reading the testimony that he gave before the Senate committee, as well as his follow-up written testimony, I am once again, struck by the fact that the behavior of FDA Commissioner Kessler and those who guide the FDA's actions are irrational and constitute a public menace.

I am also struck by the fact that bureaucrats in government, like Commissioner Kessler, can be guilty of crimes against humanity yet never have to take responsibility for their actions. Cloaked in the protection of government bureaucracy, Commissioner Kessler and his upper echelon henchmen have clearly increased the suffering of the public by blocking their access to useful information about the value of dietary supplements.

Much of that useful information is in this book. That was Dr. Janson's purpose, and he certainly accomplished it. Those who act on his sound recommendations will surely benefit—likely more than they expect.

Julian Whitaker, MD
Editor: *Health and Healing*

Introduction

Who Needs This Book and How to Use It

Who Needs This Book

If you are interested in health, and almost everybody is, this book is for you. The word "vitamins" in the title really refers to a wide variety of dietary supplements that can help you get on the road to vibrant and vital living. They can help you get well and stay well and almost certainly enhance your longevity.

If you want the most out of life and want to learn how dietary supplements can help, you will find valuable information here. You will find specific guidelines for setting up the dietary supplement part of your own health program.

If you are a physician interested in helping your patients with the latest dietary supplement therapy, you will find this a useful reference. I have drawn on my 20 years experience with supplements to direct you to the basic guidelines for this part of treatment. (Remember that dietary supplements are only a part of comprehensive medical and health management.) As you get more involved in this field, you will find that you can use fewer medications and lower doses of the ones you do use. Your patients will have fewer illnesses, and they will get well faster with supplements. If they need surgery, there will be fewer complications, and you will observe faster wound healing and shorter recovery times if they take dietary supplements.

The book includes some supplement guidelines for preventive medicine, and there are examples of treatment programs for a number of specific medical conditions. Many other health problems are also manageable with programs that include dietary supplements. This is a different way of practicing medicine, but it is gratifying to get away from technological and drug-oriented medical care when simpler and safer options are available.

If you are a researcher in the nutrition field, you may be interested to know how the results of your research are being applied in clinical practice by physicians and other health practitioners. You may also be surprised to find out that the general public is applying your scientific information to its everyday health problems and that some doctors are using your information for medical treatment instead of using drugs. You might also want to take supplements for your own health (in addition to the specific substances that you are researching).

How to Use This Book

If you want to jump into a health program, you can skip to Chapter 11, "Your Personal Supplement Program." You will find the basic recommendations for preventive medicine programs with different levels of protection, and some sample treatment programs. If you want to help manage your own medical conditions, you can combine some of the sample programs related to your health concerns with your doctor's recommendations. But remember, this information is not a substitute for medical management of diseases. It is important to have the proper diagnosis and appropriate medicine or surgery, if indicated.

Background information about dietary supplements that you may want to take (or those you are already taking) is located in the appropriate chapters on the supplements. These descriptions are based on research material and clinical experience. This information might help you or a friend design supplement programs for specific health needs.

If you want to learn about the political controversy surrounding dietary supplements, look at Chapter 13, "Dietary Supplements: Political Pressure Cooker." There, you will find out about the current situation with the United States Food and Drug Administration (FDA) and their recent rules and regulations that have made it more difficult for you to learn about the specific health value of supplements. My testimony at the Senate Committee on Labor and Human Resources hearings on the Dietary Supplement Health and Education Act is in this chapter. There is also some information on the political situation as of 1995, and some information about similar problems that proponents of dietary supplements face in Canada.

The information in this book is an integral part of the total health picture. Already nearly half of the United States population take dietary supplements at least some of the time, and many of them take supplements every day. The use of dietary supplements to promote health and treat disease is not a passing fad—it is a developing science, and you can put it to your own personal use to feel better and live longer.

Chapter 1

A Revolution in Health Care: Dietary Supplements

Your Health at Risk

Your health may be at risk if you believe the current medical and food industry myths that assert that you do not need extra vitamins and minerals if you eat properly (what is commonly called a balanced diet). For decades, this has also been the position of the US Food and Drug Administration (FDA), which appears to have had an antagonism to dietary supplements since early in its history.

As of 1995, the FDA does not even allow supplement manufacturers to use in their sales literature quotes from other governmental agencies (such as the USDA[US Department of Agriculture]) or from medical research, even if the quotation accurately and favorably portrays the value of a dietary supplement. This is a political, not a scientific, position.

If you accept this inaccurate information, you will probably be left in an average state of poor health, or what most doctors call average good health. This is the condition in which the "average" person lives. You will have the "average" profile of frequent colds and other infections, headaches, fatigue, gum disease, menstrual disturbances, anxiety, poor sleep, obesity, and accelerated aging, leading to early heart disease or common cancers and premature death. *You do not have to accept this situation.*

Changes in Medicine

Significant changes are taking place in health care. Doctors are increasingly becoming interested in the use of high-dose dietary supplements in the treatment and prevention of disease. They are, in fact, taking supplements themselves, even though they may not yet be recommending them for their patients. A recent survey showed that eight out of 10 physicians report taking vitamin E. Researchers sometimes have a curious position—for example, one researcher's studies show the value of vitamin E, but he says, "there is not enough research to recommend it to the general public, *but I am taking it myself!"* Why should you, as part of the general public, have to wait for scientists and doctors to give you the go-ahead for what they are already doing?

Recently a colleague asked me what dose of a particular nutrient I would use in a patient w th heart failure. He had tried everything else and was now willing to try a dietary supplement in the face of failure of the medical treatment. I hope that in the future he will consider using supplements before the situation is dire, so it may not get that way. Unfortunately, many mainstream practitioners worry about the ridicule of their colleagues if they consider using dietary supplements instead of the usual medication.

Dietary supplements are an integral part of a comprehensive health program. I have been taking them myself since 1971 and recommending them as part of my medical practice since 1976. When I graduated from medical school in 1970, I knew virtually nothing about the field of nutrition. At that time, a common joke was that the average physician knew as much about nutrition as the average secretary, unless the secretary had a weight problem, in which case the secretary knew more than the doctor!

Unfortunately, things in medical school haven't changed much. Most medical schools do not go into detail about nutrition during the entire 4 years of training. However, changes are just beginning in medical education, mainly due to public demand for more nutrition information and more choice of therapies. For the most part, this is not being initiated by the medical schools, but is coming primarily from physician self-education groups such as the *American College for Advancement in Medicine*, the *American Academy of Environmental Medicine* and the *American Holistic Medical Association*.

Only recently have medical schools introduced courses in "alternative medicine" or "complementary medicine." There is a demand for this information, and, once they are exposed to it, medical students often have a strong interest. Therefore, this field is likely to grow. Because hospitals and medical schools have very little experience with these health practices, some of the courses leave out many of the best-documented and most effective treatments using dietary supplements, but they are getting their feet wet.

Opponents of Change

There are some antagonists to this development in medical education and health care. They are mired in the old way of thinking about nutrition and dietary supplements. They often make the erroneous claim that the therapeutic value of dietary supplementation is not supported by scientific literature or that it is dangerous. This is simply the last gasp of a cadre of status quo protectors. They often appear to have the ulterior motive of supporting drug companies and a medical care system that needs to change. Sometimes their motives are not clear.

At a 1995 conference on nutrition controversies, sponsored by the University of Vermont, three of my research colleagues and one medical colleague spoke about the value of dietary supplements in health care. Prior to the conference, the program director received a phone call from an antagonist who threatened to call every presenter cautioning them not to speak because he disagreed with the information that we were going to present. The director was not intimidated, but one speaker with a more traditional view did withdraw. These tactics, designed to suppress debate, should not be tolerated in America.

Sometimes, antagonists to the use of dietary supplements claim that the extra nutrients only lead to "expensive urine" because extra amounts of most vitamins are excreted by the kidneys. This is irrelevant, since the important issue is not the ultimate fate of the substances, but what they do while they are on their way through the body and how many tissues they heal—including the urinary tract. In fact, a recent study showed that large doses of vitamins and minerals markedly reduced tumor recurrence in patients with bladder cancer, compared to those who received just the Recommended Dietary Allowances. This was a reputable study, published in the *Journal of Urology*!

Luckily, I was introduced to nutrition *after* medical school and was able to pursue it with an open mind. I did not have to contend with as much opposition as I would have had during medical school. Since that time, I have had to learn (and unlearn) a lot. This knowledge of nutritionally oriented health care is available in the medical literature and at conferences, through numerous books, and, perhaps most important, from clinical experience and discussions with colleagues.

It is the clinical experience with patients taking dietary supplements that acts as a filter and helps me to understand what really works. Every day I am able to observe the therapeutic and preventive benefits of dietary supplements in both my medical practice and in everyday life.

Other Health Practices

Before you get the wrong impression, you should understand that supplements are a *part* of a comprehensive health program. A total approach includes a healthy diet. I recommend that this be mostly vegetarian, whole foods, *without* added sugars, white flour, white rice, artificial colors or flavors, preservatives, margarines or other hydrogenated oils, and very little of any added oil or fat (but enough of the right oils—more about this later).

Total health also requires that you be physically active. Since most people lead relatively sedentary lives, an exercise program is essential. Begin an aerobic fitness program, such as brisk walking, cycling or running, with some stretching or yoga. Try to participate in these activities for at least 30 to 40 minutes, no fewer than three or four times per week. It is a good idea to work up a mild sweat but not to get out of breath (if you get out of breath, the exercise is not aerobic).

Coping with stress is another essential part of total health. In addition to other problems of modern life (and, I suspect, life throughout history), most people are under some degree of stress. Stress is our level of reactivity to variations from a perfect environment, whether internal or external. Stressors are the environmental variables that lead us to experience stress. A stress management program of visualization, breathing or meditation, self-regulation, biofeedback or any of a number of relaxation methods will contribute to both disease prevention and treatment. (Preventive medicine is great, but if you haven't managed to prevent everything bad, it is good to know that preventive medicine also works in the treatment of many medical conditions.)

Health and Life Extension

Both treatment and prevention of disease are the goals of these comprehensive health program recommendations. One of the side benefits of taking such good care of yourself is the likelihood of enhanced longevity. The desire for a long life is a sign of the love you have for the moment in which you are living and a sign of your love for yourself. Until you develop that self love, it is very difficult to start on the road to better health or implement the programs that will take you there.

Many people who seek health counseling come with the particular goal of extending their healthy years. There are many components to comprehensive life-extension programs, and stress reduction is a significant contributor to them. Proper diet and exercise are essential to enhanced longevity, and specific dietary supplements are also powerful contributors to achieving this goal. To be positively healthy into advanced years requires that you combine as many good health practices as possible into your personal action plan.

Having said all this, the purpose of this book is to give you the information you need to start your own dietary supplement program, usually using relatively large yet safe and effective doses, for preventing and treating both symptoms and diseases and enhancing longevity.

Diagnoses Versus Optimal Health

A diagnosis is just a name given to a recognized collection of symptoms. If your particular collection of symptoms does not fit a known pattern, they cannot be diagnosed (but that does not mean that you do not have health problems). Many doctors assume that if you do not have a clear diagnosis your symptoms are not real or that they are "all in your head." Or they may think the situation is not serious enough to require treatment. ("Come back when it gets worse, and we'll see what we can do.") This was the case with Premenstrual Syndrome before it was a recognized pattern, and it is the case today with Chronic Fatigue Syndrome, which has only recently become accepted by physicians as a "legitimate" health problem. The lack of a diagnosis does not mean you are in optimal health.

If you look hard enough, most symptoms have an underlying cause rooted in altered biochemistry and physiology. Often, these causes are related to lifestyle choices that have metabolic consequences. There are many estimates that up to 85% of such problems are the result of these choices, and many of them are related to nutrients. Most of these symptoms can be relieved without drugs or surgery, but not all of them. Knowing the difference is an important part of holistic medicine.

Nutrients and Other Supplements

There are approximately 50 known essential nutrients, including vitamins, minerals, essential fatty acids (oils), and amino acids. These nutrients must be acquired in relatively small amounts from the diet or from supplements in order to maintain minimal health and to prevent specific deficiency diseases such as pellagra, beriberi and scurvy. Deficiency diseases, however, are not the common health problems in America or the rest of the industrialized world. Marginal nutrition associated with marginal health is much more likely to be the problem for most people. You may, for example, have enough vitamin C to prevent scurvy, but not enough to have optimal health, a sense of vitality, and a vigorous immune defense.

There are also a number of "accessory food factors" that are found in food but are not essential because you can manufacture them in the body from other substances. The amount that you manufacture is sometimes inadequate for optimal health, and in these situations, supplementation is essential for treatment or prevention of illness. These accessory food factors include coenzyme Q10, L-carnitine, GLA (gamma-linolenic acid), some non-essential amino acids and other dietary supplements.

Besides all of these nutrients, there are other substances found in the food supply that are not considered essential but that, nonetheless, offer important health benefits. Many of these are bioflavonoids, or simply, flavonoids. They are plant pigments that may act as antioxidants or enhance the effects of other nutrients or physiological molecules. Some of them are also available as supplements, but there are many recently discovered ones that are not. (Let this serve as a reminder of how important it is to eat a healthy diet.)

Are Supplements Natural?

You may be thinking that it is not "natural" to take supplements. In some ways this is true, but our food supply is not as rich in nutrients as we have been led to believe, and dietary supplements are proven to be valuable for enhancing health, as well as treating and preventing illness. They are usually extra amounts of substances that we all need (except the herbs), and unlike drugs, they work by enhancing normal metabolic functions or protecting us from environmental stressors. We do not live in a natural environment. Also, everything natural is not necessarily healthy or beneficial to humans. For example, earthquakes, floods and syphilis are all "natural," but they are not desirable. Supplements can help you resist unavoidable negative influences, both natural and unnatural.

The most common view of preventive medicine is that it involves things that you shouldn't do—smoke, drink excessive alcohol, take drugs, overeat. These negatives are an essential but incomplete approach to prevention. A more positive view is that of being an active participant in your own health promotion program. Supplementing your diet is one way to actively promote your own wellness, create vitality and enhance longevity. Dietary supplements have worked for many people for many years. Take my word for it, they can work for you too.

Chapter 2

Why You Need Vitamins

Along with the many people I encounter in my medical practice and my lectures, you may wonder, "Why do I need to take supplements?" Many people think, and some conservative nutritionists would agree with them, that eating a balanced diet provides all the vitamins they need. This is simply not so. Everyone's idea of a balanced diet, even among experts, is different, and it may vary greatly from the scientifically based recommendations of a contemporary nutritionist or nutritionally oriented physician. In order to answer the question, we need to explore a number of different but equally important personal and ecological considerations: genetics, environment, agriculture, stress and health history, and of course, your desire for a vigorous and lively health future.

The Important Role of Genetics

Throughout all species there is wide variation in genetic makeup. This variation includes differing abilities to survive in a given nutritional environment. In other words, to survive well, one animal may require much more or less of particular nutrients than another animal. Dr. Roger Williams has shown in experiments with rats that after five generations of inbreeding, litter mates, which are very close genetically, can vary in nutrient needs up to 40 times for particular nutrients. In other words, one may need 2.5 mg of pantothenic acid (vitamin B5) and another may need 100 mg for the same level of vitality, physical endurance and life span. There is an even greater variation in human beings, as we have a greater genetic diversity than other species.

In the natural course of events, species develop (or evolve) when those animals with greater nutritional needs fail to survive or to reproduce as well as those with lesser needs. Except in a few known genetic disorders, we cannot determine subtle variations in nutritional needs for human beings. It is therefore wise to make sure that our internal environment (including all cells, tissues and organs) is abundantly supplied with all the nutrients. Biochemical individuality is Dr Williams' term for the basic principle of varied individual needs.

In tissue cultures (cells growing in laboratories) the culture medium is made quite rich in all the required nutrients. If the cells were only given minimum requirements, some cells would not thrive and researchers would risk losing the cell line. In human beings the blood plasma provides nourishment for the cells, and needs a constant and abundant supply of all the nutrients. This requires both a healthy diet and supplements.

Supplements enhance a healthy diet; they are not a substitute for it. Some antagonists to the use of dietary supplements have said that people will get a false sense of security if they use supplements, and as a result they will not seek out the healthiest foods. It is my experience, on the contrary, that the people who elect to use supplements are usually the ones who also eat a healthier diet. These antagonists are usually the same people who defend the highly processed, westernized, or "industrial" diet that is a prime cause of degenerative disease and chronic health problems.

Our Risky Environment

Another reason you will benefit from dietary supplements is the poor quality of the environment in which we live. Whether it is toxins in food, water, and air or other exposures such as mercury in dental fillings or aluminum in cookware and antiperspirants, our bodies have an excessive burden to overcome. This environmental burden taxes our detoxification capacity and may lead to many health problems.

You already know that the air is polluted. Everybody is subjected to toxic exposure from a wide variety of pollutants in the air they breathe. Among the many toxins in the air are:

1. Carbon monoxide and lead from fuel exhaust (most of the lead has been reduced in the United States, but it is still found elsewhere).

2. Hydrocarbon pollutants from industrial waste.

3. By-products from the burning of fossil fuels.

4. Radiation leakage from nuclear power plants and radon in the home. Radiation, like radon gas, is a contaminant that cannot be seen, smelled, or tasted and is therefore more insidious than some of the more familiar pollutants.

Tap water, unfortunately, contains more than water. It is often contaminated with toxic heavy metals such as lead or cadmium or with fluoride (associated with an increased risk of cancer, digestive disorders and kidney disease). Often, industrial chemicals and wastes, pesticides and other farm chemicals have seeped through the soil to contaminate the water table. Volatile chemicals (those hydrocarbons that readily vaporize) can combine with chlorine to form even more toxic products.

You may be familiar with the toxic chemical water con-tamination in Woburn, Massachusetts, which led to increases in childhood leukemia. Other examples abound. (I recom-mend a solid carbon-block water filter, or spring water, for all drinking and cooking needs.) Unfortunately, in spite of home filtration or spring water for personal use, there is always some exposure to tap water, such as when you eat at restaurants or buy prepared foods, or when you shower and breathe the vaporized volatile chemicals. (At one water testing lab, the joke about their municipal water was that it was "safe" to drink, but for goodness sake don't smoke in the shower!)

Cigarette smoke exposure in smokers and nonsmokers (sidestream smoke—the uninhaled pollutants from the end of the cigarette—and secondhand smoke are also highly toxic) creates further health risks. This and most pollutants lead to an increase of high-energy molecular fragments known as *free radicals*. These free radicals can severely dam-age tissues, destroy nutrients, and lead to premature aging, heart disease and cancer. All of these environmental prob-lems increase your need for nutrients, and many supple-ments can help control the damage of toxic exposures.

The Damage from Free Radicals

In the normal course of metabolism, your body pro-duces small, high-energy particles that have a single elec-tron in their outer shell (such molecules are unstable be-cause electrons prefer to be paired). These are called free radicals, and they can be very damaging in their search for another electron. Free radicals derived from oxygen are the most abundant and damaging of the species.

These free radicals are normally channeled into energy production. In some cells they may be used as the weapons to kill viruses and bacteria. Unfortunately, if too many of them are produced, their extremely high energy can also be damaging to normal tissues. Free radicals disrupt the normal production of DNA, the genetic material, and alter the lipids (fats) in cell membranes. They also affect the blood vessels and the production of prostaglandins. (Prostaglandins are hormone-like substances that regulate many physiological functions, and their production is very sensitive to many metabolic influences.)

We are also exposed to free radicals that are found in the environment or generated by exposure to environmental chemicals. There are many sources of excess free-radical exposure, including cigarette smoke; air pollution; some highly processed foods and food additives; ultraviolet sunlight and radiation; processed oils such as commercial vegetable oils, margarines and shortenings; charcoal-broiled foods and any charred or burned foods; heavy metals (lead, cadmium, aluminum, and mercury) found in processed foods; excessive iron; pesticides; and some prescription medications. Many of the chemicals found in municipal water supplies are toxic because they generate free radicals. It is good to drink a lot of water but to avoid tap water as much as possible.

Recently, it has been confirmed that excessive accumulation of iron, common in meat-eating populations, may be a highly significant risk factor in the development of heart disease, although not as important as smoking. This is probably due to this *transition metal* being a generator of free radicals. Therefore, it is also a probable risk factor for cancer. Unless you have a demonstrated need for iron, it is a good idea to avoid supplements that contain it, although these studies were *not* done with iron supplements.

By careful lifestyle choices some of these free-radical sources can be avoided and others can be counteracted. By making these choices for yourself you can slow down the aging process, decrease the risk of cancer and heart disease and promote high energy and a vital, healthy feeling of well-being. One way to protect yourself from free-radical damage is to take dietary supplements. The chapters on the individual supplements contain more specific information.

We need extra supplies of those nutrients destroyed by toxins and those that help to prevent the harmful effects of these foreign chemicals. Specifically, vitamins A, C, E and beta-carotene; the trace minerals selenium and zinc; and accessory food factors, such as bioflavonoids and coenzyme Q10, all help to scavenge free radicals through antioxidant activity. They help prevent cancer, heart disease, premature aging and tissue degeneration. Many herbs also help in the fight against excess free radicals.

Destructive Agricultural Practices

Modern agricultural practices have adversely affected the quality of our food supply. Growing foods with methods designed to increase quantity, or to facilitate transportation and storage (such as the development of sturdy, square tomatoes) is often detrimental to their nutritional value. Nutritional value is rarely considered when developers play with the genetics of plants or soil modifications.

Soil quality has been degraded through modern farming methods. Most chemical fertilizers do not replace all of the minerals needed for human nutrition. Organic foods have been shown to have a higher nutritional value than conventionally grown foods. They are also free of the pesticides, herbicides and thousands of other risky chemicals that are added to foods during processing. There is also wide variation in the natural mineral content of the soil. For example, in northeastern states (and elsewhere) the soil has a very low selenium content. Selenium is important for protection from heart disease and cancer. In spite of a diet that includes foods from many geographic areas, research has shown that people living in regions with low soil selenium have a higher risk of cancer. Although selenium, as well as chromium and iodine, are essential for human nutrition, they are not required for growing healthy plants. They are rarely added to the soil for agricultural purposes.

Foods are often picked before they are ripe and allowed to ripen in transit, at the market or during home storage. They do not acquire their full complement of minerals and vitamins, which frequently increase greatly during the later stages of growth. In addition, transportation and storage of foods, whether in the market or at home, allows time for nutrients to deteriorate. Fruits and vegetables can lose significant amounts of vitamin C after 3 days in cold storage, and even more at room temperature. Dried fruits can also lose vitamins A, C and E if exposed to oxygen and light. This is not to say that stored foods are of no value, but the lower nutrient content increases the importance of taking supplements.

You can overcome some of these problems if you grow your own food or buy organically grown fruits and vegetables (which are generally fresher because they cannot be stored as long). Commercial fruits and vegetables are frequently sprayed with toxic chemicals. Many of these substances are harmful, and they accumulate in body fat, with deleterious health effects over the years. A good example is DDT, which is still present in human fat tissue although its use was banned years ago.

Many of the pesticides prohibited in the United States have been freely sold to third world countries, which then export foods to the US. Controls on the use of pesticides and other chemicals are not strict in many of these countries. The workers who apply these chemicals frequently have diseases that are the result of their high exposures. Certain nutritional supplements can help counter the ill effects of many of these poisons. They include vitamins C, E and B complex, carotenes, bioflavonoids, and others. Of course, it is also wise to choose untreated foods as much as possible.

Stress Increases Needs

Although we seem to live in a time of great stress, I believe that this is not unique to our age. There have always been many stressors that have adversely influenced human health. Earlier generations did not have the advantage of high-dose nutrients to help diminish the toll of these stressors in their lives.

Stress, whether emotional or physical or due to injury or illness, depletes the body of nutrients, especially vitamin C, the B complex and zinc. Vitamin B6 and pantothenic acid are also particularly important in times of stress. Vitamins C and E and zinc promote the healing process. A comprehensive approach to good health includes practices that aid in stress management, regular exercise and proper diet. Diet and nutritional supplements provide the building blocks to form a healthier, more vital organism.

Health History

You may have heard of someone's grandparent who lived to a ripe old age with little attention to diet or nutritional supplements. This is quite possible. However, it is important to realize that potential human life span is well over 100 years. Living to 80 or 90 years may result from growing up with cleaner air and water, fresher food, fewer chemical exposures and lesser availability of highly processed foods. Also, many people who survive a long time have numerous health problems. In spite of these occasional reports of decadent oldsters, we are seeing more frequent and earlier degenerative diseases. Remember, the quality of life is more important than the quantity. Dietary supplements can promote what most of us would prefer— good health and vigor in all stages of life, including later years.

There is great individual genetic variation. You may have inherited a strong constitution, but is it really wise to wait 40 or 50 years to find out? Nutritional supplements help people who have greater genetically determined needs to remain vigorous and active well into old age. Many poor health habits, such as consumption of sweets, alcohol, caffeine, highly processed foods and artificial food additives, lack of exercise and high stress, increase nutrient needs. The typical American diet is a sad joke. It would be hard to design a diet that could do more harm to health than the one most Americans eat every day.

Stress reduction and relaxation techniques, body therapies and exercise programs are part of good health, but nutritional supplementation is extremely important to the comprehensive approach to health care and preventive medicine. Specific chronic and acute illnesses can be treated with large doses of nutrient supplements. They can usually reduce or eliminate the need for drugs or surgery.

Your Health Future

After considering all these issues, the last and perhaps most important point is that your future health depends on a number of your current health practices—which you have the power to change. Taking dietary supplements of any kind will almost certainly help you overcome many of your current health problems and enhance your energy. And they will protect you from disease and degeneration well into a vital, vigorous, and healthy future.

A Note on the RDAs

The Recommended Dietary Allowances are established by the Food and Nutrition Board of the National Research Council, National Academy of Science. These nutrient levels are supposed to prevent deficiency diseases in most healthy people. Unfortunately, the values have been heavily influenced by the food industry, economic considerations and politics, not just by science.

Many researchers question the value of the RDAs. They make the highly processed American food supply look more nutritious than it is, and they appear to be influenced by the food industry. The RDAs are *not* useful in establishing *optimal* health. You are at little risk of developing the deficiency diseases—pellagra, scurvy, or beriberi. Our modern problems are not deficiency diseases but degenerative diseases. Nutrients play an important role in preventing these conditions. The RDAs cannot be used in evaluating the therapeutic and preventive value of large doses of dietary supplements.

The sad truth is, if you look around, you will see many people who do manage to get the RDA levels of most nutrients, but they still go on to develop early heart disease, cancer, arthritis, and diabetes. They have frequent viral infections (colds, the flu, herpes), they are overweight, and they lose their teeth to decay and gum disease. In terms of life expectancy, infant mortality and health care costs, Americans are not in the most favorable position in world statistics. Average Americans have a lower life expectancy than citizens of some third world countries.

In this regard, it is not good to be average—the average American will die early of heart disease, stroke, diabetes or cancer. You can do many things to improve your health and reduce your risk of developing the health problems of the rest of the population. Taking dietary supplements is one of them. And it is an important one. Let's explore what nutrients may do for your health, energy and general sense of vitality and well-being.

Chapter 3

'Orthomolecular' Medicine: The Right Molecules in the Right Amounts

Orthomolecular medicine is the restoration and maintenance of health through the administration of adequate amounts of substances that are normally present in the body. "Ortho" means correct, and "molecular" means, well, molecular. Thus, orthomolecular medicine simply refers to creating the correct molecular balance in the body. This definition of orthomolecular medicine was established by Linus Pauling in 1968 to describe more accurately what had been called "megavitamin therapy."

Orthomolecular treatment had been used first in the early 1950s by Drs. Abram Hoffer and Humphrey Osmond for the treatment of mental illness. The success rate varied, but high doses of niacin (vitamin B3) helped a significant number of their patients with schizophrenia. Vitamin C, pyridoxine (vitamin B6), magnesium and zinc were later added to typical orthomolecular programs for the treatment of mental illness. Interestingly, Hoffer and Osmond did these first "double-blind" studies in psychiatry before the advent of the phenothiazine drugs (such as Thorazine®,

Stelazine®, Mellaril®, Prolixin®, and Haldol®), which since then have become the foundation of mainstream psychiatric treatment.

The substances used in orthomolecular medicine may be nutrients or molecules manufactured in the body, such as hormones, or the accessory food factors referred to above. Orthomolecular physicians are more cautious in their use of hormone supplements, such as DHEA, thyroid or melatonin, because of their potent effects and sometimes greater risk of side effects compared with vitamins and minerals. (DHEA and melatonin have been shown to be quite safe even in very large doses; usually natural hormones are much safer than the synthetics that are commonly used in medicine, except for melatonin.) They will frequently use some herbs and other natural products for treatment whenever they provide margins of safety and effectiveness that are significantly better than medications—which is usual.

Do No Harm

The first principle of medical ethics is "Do no harm." Unfortunately, the bulk of medical practice today is based on drug therapy and surgery, which are frequently harmful, although sometimes necessary. The sad fact is that more people die in any one year from the side effects of prescribed medication than from car accidents, and this is when the drugs are taken as directed. For most nutritional supplements, the doses used for treatment and prevention are far removed from the doses that may be harmful. In fact, only a few of them have any potential toxicity. Vitamin C, for example, can be and has been taken in enormous doses (over 80–100 g) without significant side effects. No matter how much vitamin C you take, it is probably safer than the water with which you take it.

My colleague Alan Gaby, MD, stated the situation elegantly in his book, *B6 The Natural Healer* (Keats Publishing, 1987): "We are grateful to modern medical science for what it has given us. Antibiotics, hormones, new surgical techniques, and advanced diagnostic devices have saved many lives. Yet, medicine as it is practiced today is too expensive, too dangerous, and too often ineffective. The evidence continues to mount that diet and nutrient therapy can be a safe, effective, and inexpensive alternative to drugs and surgery."

Potent Substances

Dietary supplements are potent substances. Microscopic amounts can prevent deficiency diseases, and larger amounts may be therapeutic. Some health problems are chronic, nagging symptoms that may be relieved temporarily by medicine, only to recur when your susceptibility is high. Common examples are allergies, eczema, headaches, hypoglycemia, digestive upset, anxiety, acne, fatigue, arthritis, sinusitis and asthma (which may be more severe). These illnesses are not usually lethal, but they can make your life miserable. Most medical therapies do not deal with them effectively or prevent their recurrence.

Other health problems are more serious. It is estimated that 85% of the chronic, degenerative diseases that kill people are related to lifestyle choices. These include heart disease, diabetes, cancer and strokes. The lifestyle choices that influence them are diet, smoking, alcohol, non-therapeutic drugs, caffeine consumption, exercise, nutrient supplements and stress reduction.

Dietary supplements have a strong effect on the development and relief of all of these uncomfortable or life-threatening problems. They can both relieve symptoms and prevent relapse. They can also reduce the incidence and risk of dying from the potentially lethal diseases such as heart disease, diabetes and cancer. I have been saying this for 20 years, based on literature reports that were definitive or strongly suggestive, and on the long safety record of dietary supplements.

Prevention and Treatment

In the past few years, more and more studies have been confirming the view that nutrients are therapeutic and preventive. Vitamin C, vitamin E, beta-carotene, selenium, zinc, and magnesium are among the many nutrients that have been shown to contribute positively to health and longevity. Even the National Cancer Institute is looking more favorably on vitamin C these days, especially due to the work of Dr. Linus Pauling. I was surprised to see an article several years ago in the prestigious *New England Journal of Medicine*, written by researcher Dr. Mark Levine, on the biology and biochemistry of vitamin C, suggesting that the RDA might not be adequate for optimal health. This idea was revolutionary for the mainstream medical press.

Vitamins are generally defined as complex organic substances that are essential in the diet because they are not manufactured in the body, yet they participate in physiological reactions. The definition is not quite precise, because some substances, such as vitamin D, are produced in the body, although not necessarily in adequate quantities. Also, the body produces vitamin A from beta-carotene, which is (incorrectly) called a provitamin. Some substances are not exactly vitamins, but they are like vitamins because they are part of other nutrients, such as para-aminobenzoic acid (PABA), choline and inositol.

I have been taking dietary supplements for 25 years. I take a wide variety of vitamins, minerals, amino acids, flavonoids and herbs. I usually take large doses of the most protective nutrients—I will tell you more about what I take later. You, too, can be a part of this health revolution. Making informed choices of dietary supplements in combination with a healthy diet, exercise and stress management will have a positive influence on your life.

In the next chapters, you will find an explanation of many of the health benefits of specific dietary supplements that I have found helpful in my holistic medical practice. Large doses of many of these substances have been shown to lower cholesterol, decrease blood pressure, enhance immunity and resistance to infection, decrease the risk of cancer, slow the aging process, increase energy and stamina, improve sugar regulation, and restore healthy gum tissue. They also reduce the incidence of birth defects and miscarriage. They can probably help you reduce your frequency of colds and other infections, decrease allergy symptoms, improve energy levels and enhance your general sense of well being. As you will see, these are only some of the reasons to take many of these dietary supplements.

All of the substances described as antioxidants or free-radical scavengers help to slow the aging process; reduce the risk of cancer and heart disease; decrease skin wrinkling due to sun exposure, smoking or age; detoxify environmental pollutants including cigarette smoke; decrease the production of age pigment in the skin ("liver spots" or "age spots"); and protect you from the damaging effects of X-rays and ultraviolet light. Supplements as well as rich nutritional food sources are essential to reduce your risk of degenerative diseases and give you the best chance of living a long and healthy life.

All comprehensive health programs require more than nutrient supplements. When I design health programs, I use a health and medical history, laboratory tests and educated intuition based on many years of experience, scientific literature and discussions with colleagues who also have years of experience using dietary supplements.

Supplements are not only useful in the prevention of illness and maintenance of a positive state of health, but many of them are also valuable in the treatment of specific medical conditions. *However, none of these descriptions of the clinical usefulness of supplements is meant to serve as a prescription or as medical treatment without consultation with a health practitioner.* These are some of the clinical applications of nutrients that are reasonably well supported in the medical literature and have helped patients in my experience, but these specific combinations may not be appropriate for you.

Nutrients and Herbs

There are many substances that are clinically useful in physiological approaches to health care and preventive medicine. They are sometimes referred to by the generic term "vitamins," but they include vitamins, minerals, amino acids, essential fatty acids and natural hormones. There are also conditionally essential nutrients (those that are necessary in some circumstances, such as coenzyme Q10 and L-carnitine) and accessory food factors (such as flavonoids), which have physiological functions but are not essential in the diet as far as we know.

In addition to these nutrients, there are natural therapeutic herbs and plant extracts from various traditional healing cultures, such as Chinese, Indian and Native American herbs. Technically, because herbs usually contain substances that are not normally present in the body, they are not part of orthomolecular medicine, but they are usually helpful in the healing process and have low or no known toxicity. It is impossible to include all therapeutic herbs here. I have included some of those I have found most useful in my practice.

This is not a comprehensive list of all the therapeutic uses of the products described, but it is a summary of the most important health relationships that I have found in clinical practice over the last 20 years. It would be wise to consult a professional for individual advice, especially if you have unusual health or medical needs. It is also a good idea to do a lot of self-education. Don't forget to include diet, exercise, stress management and personal development as part of your comprehensive health plan.

Multivitamin/Mineral Supplements

It makes supplement programs much easier if you start out with a high-quality multivitamin/mineral combination. In these descriptions of how to take individual supplements, the basic recommended amounts for many of them will usually be found in such a multi, and you will probably need to take from four to eight tablets per day to get those doses. Sometimes the amount in the multi is adequate for most health needs if you do not want to take too many pills, but usually a number of additional supplements will enhance your health program.

The multivitamin/mineral that I use in my office is a comprehensive professional formulation. Many nutritionally oriented physicians will use comparable formulas, and there are similar ones available from both retail health food stores and some mail-order sources. The following content list is the total that you will find in *six tablets* (the daily recommendation) of this particular formula. For convenience, it is called *Basic Multiple* in the next chapters. Check if your multi has similar figures, and it will make supplementing your diet much easier. If it is slightly different, it may be of only minor significance. Striking differences can usually be made up with a few additional supplements.

The formula for six daily tablets of the *Basic Multiple:*

Vitamin A	10,000 IU
Vitamin C	1,200 mg
Beta-carotene	15,000 IU
Vitamin D3	400 IU
Vitamin E (*d*-alpha+mixed)	400 IU
Thiamine (B1)	100 mg
Riboflavin (B2)	50 mg
Niacinamide (B3)	150 mg
Niacin (B3)	40 mg
Pyridoxine (B6)	100 mg
Folate (folic acid)	800 mcg
Vitamin B12	100 mcg
Biotin	300 mcg
Pantothenic acid	500 mg
Calcium	500 mg
Magnesium	500 mg
Iodine	200 mcg
Zinc	30 mg
Selenium	200 mcg
Chromium	200 mcg
Copper	3 mg
Manganese	20 mg
Molybdenum	100 mcg
Potassium	99 mg
Choline	150 mg
Citrus bioflavonoids	100 mg
PABA	50 mg
Vanadium	50 mcg
Boron	3 mg

L- and N-acetyl-cysteine .... 200 mg
Methionine .... 62.5 mg
Glutamic HCl .... 25 mg
Betaine HCl .... 150 mg

This *Basic Multiple* formula has the right balance of major nutrients in the essential quantities for basic good health. Calcium:magnesium ratios may vary somewhat in multiples from different sources. There are several variations of this formula (such as with iron or without copper) for special needs. In order to meet your individual needs, any multi that you choose should have that flexibility. Adjustment of specific nutrient doses is easy with additional supplements, beyond what is contained in any one multiple. Remember that these nutrients are meant to be in addition to what you will obtain from your diet.

Units and Measurements

It may help you to have some explanations of dosage terminology before I describe the individual nutrients. A kilogram (kg) is a metric measure of weight equivalent to approximately 2.2 pounds, while a gram (g) is 1/1000 of a kilogram. A milligram (mg) is 1/1000 of a gram, and a microgram (mcg) is 1/1000 of a milligram.

International units, or IU, are different for each nutrient. For example for vitamin E they are determined with reference to biological activity in maintaining pregnancy in rats. One *milli*gram is approximately 1.49 IU of natural vitamin E. For vitamin A, IU are measured in "retinol equivalents" and 1 *micro*gram is approximately 5 IU.

It is important not to make a mistake when reading units and weights, both for safety and for being sure you are getting what you are paying for. Read labels carefully and review this information, if necessary.

Nutrient Classifications

One way of classifying vitamins is by whether they are fat or water soluble. The fat-soluble vitamins are vitamin A, beta-carotene, and vitamins D, E, and K. Coenzyme Q10 is another fat-soluble nutrient, although it is not, strictly speaking, a vitamin. Essential fatty acids are obviously fat soluble, but they are worthy of their own discussion. Certain substances, such as mineral oil, some medications, and excesses of certain fibers in the diet may reduce the absorption of fat-soluble nutrients or some minerals.

One property of some of the fat-soluble nutrients is that they may be readily stored either in fatty tissue or in the liver. Vitamins A and D are known to have some toxicity as a result of accumulation of large amounts, so you need to be somewhat careful of the doses that you take. It is common for the general press and supplement antagonists to exaggerate the toxicity of these nutrients, but the usual doses are quite safe. If you take very large doses for prolonged periods, you do put yourself at some risk. The usual side effects are readily reversible, but some calcifications that can result from excess vitamin D may not be.

In spite of their being fat soluble, vitamin E and coenzyme Q10 are not stored excessively, and they are readily used up in performing their protective roles. There is no known toxicity from these nutrients at any of the doses that have been studied.

The B vitamins and vitamin C are water soluble. Water-soluble nutrients have a reputation of being quite safe in almost any doses because they are not stored in the body (except for vitamin B12, which is stored in the liver but is still not toxic). For the most part, any excess intake is readily excreted in the urine. This reputation for safety is *almost* entirely deserved, but not quite. There are a few problems from excessive doses of vitamin B3 (niacin), especially in the timed-release form, and vitamin B6 (pyridoxine). The doses required for such side effects are usually enormous compared with typical therapeutic levels. The side effects have usually been completely reversible. It is wise to be aware of these risks but not overly anxious about them.

The minerals, amino acids, accessory food factors and flavonoids are not generally classified according to solubility. There are also many therapeutic herbs/botanicals and some miscellaneous substances that are valuable in health care. At the end of each supplement description, there is a brief explanation of how to take it, and in what forms it is most conveniently available.

If you have significant health problems, you need to be aware of the value of good professional medical care, and you should seek such advice. If you can find a physician in your area who understands nutritional therapy and might use it instead of medication, so much the better. If not, perhaps you can introduce your physician to these concepts. See the resources in Appendix 2 for ways to find nutritionally oriented physicians.

This explanation of dietary supplements is meant to be brief, but it should give you enough information to know what supplements to take and in what amounts for general good health and vitality. It is not a textbook or a research paper, and it is not a medical prescription.

Now, on to the supplements.

Chapter 4

Fat-Soluble Nutrients

Vitamin A

This vitamin helps you to maintain the quality of your mucous membranes and to resist infections. Vitamin A is essential for normal vision, bone growth, reproduction, and white blood cell development. It is also essential for normal immune function and fertility. It is found naturally only in animal products, but it can be made by the body from beta-carotene. The conversion from beta-carotene is an enzymatic reaction in the intestines, and this process may be sluggish. Therefore, in certain situations, it may be beneficial to take the preformed vitamin A, instead of depending on the conversion. It helps to protect the membranes from the effects of pollutants such as cigarette smoke and car exhaust. It is also useful in skin conditions such as acne. Vitamin A has some activity as an antioxidant, but not as much as beta-carotene.

Although large doses of vitamin A are *potentially toxic*, there is a fairly wide margin of safety in adults. However, I recommend that you avoid taking very large doses (over 50,000–100,000 IU) without first consulting your health practitioner. Avoid doses above 10,000 IU during the first 3 months of pregnancy. Sometimes the larger doses are used therapeutically for a short time, and some physicians use massive doses for cancer patients.

How to take

Vitamin A is commonly available in 10,000- and 25,000-IU capsules and in multivitamins. The *Basic Multiple* formula contains 10,000 IU. When I recommend extra, I usually suggest one capsule of 25,000 IU. I then adjust the dose depending on the clinical situation.

Carotenes

Beta-carotene, alpha-carotene, lutein, lycopene, zeaxanthin, and other carotenes provide some of the color in green, yellow and orange fruits and vegetables. Carotenes are highly effective antioxidants, even in tissues where oxygen levels are low. Some of the beta-carotene is converted in the body into vitamin A, but it apparently has activity independent of vitamin A. The body has a feedback mechanism that protects it from excess conversion into vitamin A, so that you have no worries about toxicity from carotenes.

A large body of scientific research shows that carotenes help protect against cancer and heart disease and the degeneration from free radicals. In some animal studies, they have even led to the regression of some cancers. High amounts as supplements or from food can lead to deposits in the subcutaneous fat and make your skin appear orange. This is a harmless condition known as carotenemia. In fact, this slightly yellow-orange skin color is a good sign, indicating that you have some extra protection from the powerful oxygen-generated free radicals.

How to take

Carotenes are usually available as 25,000-IU capsules. The synthetic beta-carotene is possibly not as effective as natural mixed carotenes. I suggest 25,000 IU in addition to the 15,000 IU that is in *Basic Multiple,* and extra for cancer patients. For people exposed to carcinogens or tobacco smoke, I recommend only natural sources to avoid the unproven but possible adverse interactions with the synthetic.

Vitamin E

Natural vitamin E (as *d*-alpha tocopherol plus the mixed tocopherols—beta, gamma and delta) is a good biological antioxidant, protecting you from the ravages of free-radical pathology, heart disease, cancer, and aging. Synthetic vitamin E (*dl*-alpha) is about 50% less active than the natural form. Be careful when reading the label, as that little "*l*" after the "*d*" may be obscure. The forms other than alpha are not used to characterize the potency of the capsules of vitamin E, but they are active, and the gamma form may be at least as important as the alpha.

Vitamin E is found naturally in plant oils, such as seeds, nuts and grains, and also in some green vegetables. Almonds are a particularly rich source, but in order to get the healthiest amounts of vitamin E it would be necessary to eat too much fat in the diet. Vitamin E is also found in natural vegetable oils, but commercial processing eliminates much of the vitamin from the end product. Extra oil in the diet (not a good idea) increases the need for vitamin E. Poor fat digestion or absorption can reduce the amount that actually gets into your bloodstream from foods.

Vitamin E helps maintain healthy circulation in the coronary arteries and peripheral blood vessels. In fact, blood levels of vitamin E are more than twice as predictive of heart disease risk as cholesterol levels (high levels of vitamin E mean lower incidence of heart disease). It can relieve exercise-induced leg or heart pain by improving the efficiency of oxygen use. Vitamin E also decreases platelet stickiness, which reduces excessive blood clotting, thereby offering protection from thrombosis, or sudden blockage of an artery. It can also lower total blood cholesterol levels, while it helps to raise the good cholesterol known as HDL (high-density lipoprotein). In the oxidized state, the so-called bad cholesterol, or LDL (low-density lipoprotein), is damaging to the arterial lining, and vitamin E can prevent the oxidation of this LDL, thereby protecting arteries from atherosclerosis.

It can help with leg cramps including those that occur at night, and also with premenstrual cramps. In many women, vitamin E can reverse fibrocystic breast disease (but you may also need to give up all caffeine if this is your problem).

Doses of 800 IU per day of vitamin E enhance immune function in the elderly by increasing the activity of the white blood cells (destroying viruses and bacteria) and by increasing antibody production. This leads to higher resistance and results in fewer infections. This is particularly important since the elderly are frequently more susceptible to infections. Vitamin E can also relieve menopausal hot flashes, although sometimes fairly high doses are necessary.

Tocopherols are necessary for normal neurologic function, and they protect against environmental toxins and peroxidation of the lipids (fats) in cell membranes. (Peroxidation is the addition of excess oxygen to molecules and is the same process responsible for rancidity of foods.) This peroxidation leads to the formation of free radicals, which hasten the aging process and cause damage to the skin and blood vessels.

As an antioxidant, vitamin E works intimately with other antioxidants and free-radical scavengers such as selenium, glutathione, carotenes, and vitamin C. This is one example of how nutrients work synergistically to have effects that are greater than those obtained when the substances are taken separately. Vitamin E also protects dietary essential fatty acids from oxidation.

How to take

The usual preventive and therapeutic doses that I use range from 400 to 1200 IU per day, but in some cases patients may need 2000 IU or more. There is no known toxicity at these doses. I always give patients 400 IU in the *Basic Multiple* and usually an additional 400 IU or 800 IU if they are elderly or have blood vessel diseases. For menopausal hot flashes I sometimes recommend up to 2000 IU per day, but with proper diet, other nutrient supplements and hormonal balance, such high doses are not usually needed. It is not possible, from diet alone, to consume adequate amounts of vitamin E for optimal health. For the full protection vitamin E has to offer, you must take supplements.

Vitamin D

Vitamin D3 (cholecalciferol) is required for normal calcium absorption, balance and utilization. It works with parathyroid hormone to maintain normal blood levels of calcium. It is essential for bone formation and maintenance and for those nerve and cell functions that depend on calcium. Vitamin D is produced in the body (and therefore it is not a true vitamin) by the action of ultraviolet light from the sun on the cholesterol in the skin. For this reason it has been called the "sunshine" vitamin, but it is really more like a steroid hormone than a vitamin. As we age, our ability to produce vitamin D in the skin declines, and our ability to absorb it is reduced. It is common for older people to have less exposure to the sun and poorer intestinal absorption.

The conversion of vitamin D to its more active metabolites takes place in the kidneys. In liver or kidney impairment, or bowel disorders, supplements of vitamin D may be necessary. Although dairy products contain added vitamin D, it is the synthetic form, or vitamin D2 (irradiated ergosterol), that is usually used.

High levels of vitamin D are potentially toxic, leading to excessive calcification of the tissues. For people consuming a lot of dairy products and processed fortified foods (which I do not recommend), they may get more than enough vitamin D. The tissue calcifications from excess vitamin D are often irreversible. It is therefore important to be careful about overdoing supplements, especially if you are unwilling to eliminate processed foods from your diet. However, moderate supplements of this nutrient, especially for the elderly, are valuable to maintain proper calcium balance.

How to take

The *Basic Multiple* formula (and many common multis on the market) contains 400 IU of vitamin D. I usually do not use more than this amount. Supplement capsules with 400 IU are available, usually mixed with vitamin A. Fish liver oils are another common source of vitamin D supplements. They are available as liquids or capsules, and they vary in their A and D content.

Coenzyme Q10

Coenzyme Q10 (CoQ10) is not a vitamin, but it is a fat-soluble antioxidant nutrient, sometimes called ubiquinone, which is normally produced in the body. However, there are circumstances in which the production is inadequate for optimal health. CoQ10 is essential for the production of ATP (adenosine triphosphate) in the little cellular engines called mitochondria. ATP is the molecule that our cells use to store energy.

With both age and illness, the production of CoQ10 declines. Especially after the age of 40, our tissue levels of

CoQ10 are markedly lower. Supplements can prevent and treat a variety of conditions, including heart disease, hypertension, rheumatic valvular disease and arrhythmias. Coenzyme Q10 supplements reduce angina (heart pain) and increase exercise tolerance. In people with congestive heart failure, it can improve the strength of the heart muscle and reduce shortness of breath. Some patients who had been told by their doctors that they needed a heart transplant because of the severity of their heart disease have improved so dramatically with CoQ10 supplements that they have been able to avoid surgery and to resume many of their normal activities.

Coenzyme Q10 also stimulates normal immune function, and it helps people with chronic fatigue syndrome and other immune system disorders. It reduces inflammation of the gums (gingivitis)—one of its earliest described therapeutic uses. CoQ10 stabilizes cell membranes, improves sugar metabolism in diabetes, improves metabolic rate and slows the aging process. It may be very helpful in patients with multiple allergies and environmental illness.

Because coenzyme Q10, like a number of other nutrients, helps so many problems, it also sometimes seems like a miracle cure. This appears to be the case only when one does not understand the physiology behind its many health benefits.

How to take

The usual therapeutically effective dose of coenzyme Q10 is 50–150 mg per day, although higher doses are often helpful in more severe heart disease. Recent reports suggest that those higher doses (200–400 mg) may also aid in the treatment of cancer, immune dysfunction and chronic fatigue syndrome. It is clear that supplements significantly increase the blood and tissue levels of coenzyme Q10.

Although CoQ10 is fat soluble, it is not toxic and does not accumulate excessively in the tissues. It is important to take it with food or in a chewable tablet containing some oils for best absorption. It is usually available in capsules containing 30–50 mg, or in chewable tablets that contain up to 100–200 mg of CoQ10, usually mixed with some lecithin to enhance absorption. There is chewable CoQ10 on the market containing some synthetic vitamin E in the base. Although synthetic vitamin E is not harmful and does have antioxidant value, I prefer the natural form.

I usually recommend 50–100 mg per day for people who have immune system disorders or fatigue, or if they are over 40 years old, when production of CoQ10 is significantly lower. If they have heart problems or cancer, I usually use higher doses, ranging from 100 to 300 mg per day, and sometimes even more.

Vitamin K

Although I have not used vitamin K as a supplement, some of my colleagues do, and it is worth mentioning. It occurs naturally in two fat-soluble forms—phylloquinone, from plants (leafy green vegetables), and menaquinone produced by your own friendly intestinal bacteria. (Menadione is a water-soluble synthetic substitute.)

Vitamin K is essential for normal blood clotting and normal bone formation. Deficiency is not usually a problem because of intestinal bacterial production. However, with various bowel diseases there may be inadequate production, and with fat malabsorption dietary sources may be inadequately absorbed. With antibiotic therapy, the intestinal bacterial source may be reduced to zero.

There are a few possible therapeutic uses for a supplement of vitamin K. In deficiencies that result from bowel inflammation or antibiotic treatment, vitamin K can restore normal blood clotting. For patients taking anticlotting medications, taking vitamin K can interfere with the actions of the medication. Do not take vitamin K supplements without medical advice in these situations. When administered with extra vitamin C, it can relieve morning sickness in pregnancy, at a dose of 5 mg per day. Finally, it may help relieve inflammation and arthritis.

Chapter 5

Water-Soluble Nutrients

Vitamin C

Vitamin C, technically ascorbic acid or ascorbate, is one of the most important nutrients. It is also one of the most remarkable substances in biology, having unique effects on the basic properties of molecules, cells and tissues. Most animals make their own vitamin C, and they can make huge amounts (especially compared to the RDA!). A goat, for example, can make 13,000 mg of vitamin C in one day, and more if it is under stress.

Ascorbic acid gets it name from the fact that it cures scurvy. It has been known for over 400 years that citrus fruits cure scurvy, but it took over 200 years and another scientific study before the British navy routinely provided this easy cure to its sailors. (The study by James Lind that led to this change was done on only nine sailors, but the results could not have been better, even if it had been a large-scale, double-blind, placebo-controlled trial. No responsible professional in this field is at all opposed to such necessary research studies, but we recognize that there are also other ways to acquire knowledge.) It is from this practice of providing citrus fruit to the navy that, even to this day, British people are called limeys. Albert Szent-Györgyi discovered and extracted the active substance from fruits and vegetables in the 1920s.

Vitamin C was popularized by Dr. Linus Pauling, a brilliant chemist, two-time Nobel Prize winner, and researcher in a wide range of scientific subjects. He wrote a book called *Vitamin C and the Common Cold*, followed by a second book called *Vitamin C, the Common Cold and the Flu*. In both books he cited the research and presented a compelling argument supporting the relationship of high doses of vitamin C to reduced viral symptoms. He subsequently collaborated with Dr. Ewan Cameron on a study showing benefits to cancer patients from vitamin C in doses of 10 g per day. Their patients had fewer symptoms and greater longevity with supplements, compared with matched controls. Pauling and Cameron wrote a book about this called *Cancer and Vitamin C*. The National Cancer Institute only recently began taking this important information seriously.

Vitamin C has a wide range of metabolic functions. It is an excellent biological antioxidant, offering protection from oxidative free-radical damage. It is essential for the production of collagen, which is the connective tissue that holds us together. Without adequate collagen production, we would literally fall apart. In fact, the early symptoms of scurvy, easy bruising and bleeding gums, which are the signs of deteriorating connective tissue, are the result of poor collagen production.

As a result of both its role in collagen strength and its antioxidant activity, vitamin C reduces the wrinkling and sagging of the skin that occurs with aging. Vitamin C also helps maintain mucous membranes, and it is essential for the production of the adrenal gland hormones, which are readily depleted in times of stress.

Vitamin C promotes immune function, partly by enhancing interferon production. Interferon is the natural antiviral substance that your cells produce when you are infected with a virus. Interferon is now available as a very expensive medication, but one of the best ways to increase your interferon is to take supplements of vitamin C.

Ascorbic acid also helps immunity by increasing two different activities of your white blood cells. Some varieties of these cells produce protective antibodies (humoral immunity) and other white cells eat bacteria and viruses (cellular immunity—not appetizing, but it can keep you healthy). Vitamin C promotes both of these functions, and also helps to detoxify environmental pollutants.

It is interesting that during an infection, the level of vitamin C in the white blood cells drops precipitously. This is just when they need it the most! When supplements of 200 mg per day are administered, very little happens to the ascorbate level in the cells. Only when 6000 mg per day are given does the level stay above normal, giving the cells a better chance to fight the infection.

In addition to enhancing interferon production, ascorbate also has its own antiviral properties, having been shown to kill some viruses if the tissue concentration is high enough. This is probably the basis for the successful use of intravenous vitamin C for viral illnesses such as hepatitis, mononucleosis and influenza.

Even taken orally in adequate doses, vitamin C reduces the symptoms of colds and other infections, including hepatitis, mononucleosis and flu. Giving high doses of ascorbate intravenously is often necessary to adequately raise tissue levels for the treatment of infections. Large oral doses, even up to 20–30 g or more, or intravenous treatment with vitamin C, can help with chronic fatigue syndrome, autoimmune disorders, multiple or severe allergies, and asthma. Asthma patients can increase their exercise tolerance by taking vitamin C before beginning exercise. Usually, 1 g taken about a half hour before exercise reduces or eliminates wheezing.

Ascorbate also helps with environmental illness related to exposure to toxic chemicals. Some patients with "Gulf War syndrome" have benefited from high doses of vitamin C (and other supplements), both orally and intravenously.

If you take too much vitamin C, the only potential untoward reaction is slightly loose bowels or even diarrhea, an indication that you need to reduce the dose a little. Actually, some people use this property of vitamin C to help relieve their constipation, but in addition to vitamin C, this usually requires a high-fiber diet and adequate fluid intake.

In certain conditions, such as severe infections or inflammations, you may need extra ascorbate intravenously for adequate therapeutic effects. This route of administration avoids any potential loosening of the bowels. *There are no other known side effects.*

There are no ascorbate-related problems with kidney stones or the destruction of vitamin B12, as has been claimed by some vitamin antagonists. The claims that vitamin C has potential risks is not supported by scientific literature. Several flawed studies suggested possible theoretical side effects, but these were contradicted by other studies and have never been shown to relate to clinical effects. If I were isolated on a desert island and could only have one vitamin supplement, it would be vitamin C (although I would really like to take vitamin E as my second choice and, perhaps, some coenzyme Q10, and please, couldn't I just take a few others also?).

How to take

Vitamin C as ascorbic acid is available in tablet, capsule or powder form. It is usually more convenient to take two or three tablets of 1000 mg each, twice per day. If you prefer, the powder is easily dissolved in water or dilute juice; a *quarter* teaspoon usually equals approximately 1000 mg. Ascorbic acid powder has a tart taste, and when added to dilute juice, makes the juice taste more like lemonade. For higher doses, the powder is easier to use (and cheaper). All these amounts are in addition to the 1200 mg in *Basic Multiple*.

Buffered vitamin C is available if you do not like the sour taste of the ascorbic acid form. The buffered form has just over 1000 mg per *half* teaspoon. Remember to rinse your mouth afterward, so the acid does not stay for long on the tooth enamel, where it might cause some erosion. The buffered vitamin C contains more minerals and less vitamin C per teaspoon than plain vitamin C powder and is usually far more expensive.

Bioflavonoids are frequently added to some of the vitamin C tablets on the market. Although they do enhance the effectiveness of vitamin C, it is usually cheaper and more effective to take the flavonoids separately in order to have flexibility in adjusting the doses individually. (More on the flavonoids later.)

A form of vitamin C called Ester-C® has been heavily marketed for several years. Dr. Pauling evaluated this product, and in his opinion there was not good evidence that it provided extra benefits. He noted that it is quite a bit more expensive than the usual sources of ascorbate. In at least one research study, Ester-C® has been shown to be inferior to plain ascorbic acid or ascorbate mixed with bioflavonoids.

B-Complex Vitamins

There are quite a few B vitamins. Most are numbered (thiamine = B1; riboflavin = B2; niacin or niacinamide = B3; pantothenate = B5; pyridoxine = B6; cobalamin = B12) but folic acid is not. Several other nutrients are sometimes considered part of the B complex, such as choline, inositol, biotin, lipoic acid, para-aminobenzoic acid and dimethyl glycine. The B vitamins have a variety of functions, and they frequently work together. It was thought at one time that you had to take equal amounts of all the B vitamins to be balanced. This is not quite true, since some people need different amounts of each one for their particular metabolism, and high doses of individual B vitamins may be therapeutic for specific conditions.

Brief examples of the therapeutic use of some of the B complex include the treatment of carpal tunnel syndrome and PMS with pyridoxine (B6) and the treatment of mental illness and high cholesterol levels with niacin (B3). You might be interested to know that this treatment of high cholesterol with high doses of niacin is one of the few ortho-molecular treatments accepted by orthodox medicine (of course, they don't call it orthomolecular).

Having regular injections of vitamin B12 is the proper treatment of pernicious anemia (anemia due to poor absorption of B12), but such doses given weekly or monthly can also help many patients with fatigue and depression, even when a deficiency cannot be demonstrated. As people age, they have great difficulty absorbing B12, and if they have poor digestion, this compounds the problem. Since B12 is not well absorbed orally, it is usually necessary to give injections for therapeutic effect, although there are some oral supplements of 1000 mcg (the ones that are intended to be dissolved in the mouth) that have helped some of my patients. B12 is one of the supplements that can lower homocysteine levels, thus reducing your risk of developing heart disease. (See pyridoxine.)

Vitamin B2 (riboflavin) is important for the maintenance of adequate antioxidant enzyme levels. It helps with cataract prevention, muscle cramps and immune function. I usually suggest only the 50 mg that is in *Basic Multiple*. It is riboflavin that gives the urine its intense yellow color when any leftover is excreted. This is a harmless situation.

Thiamin (Vitamin B1)

Thiamin is a water-soluble vitamin essential in energy metabolism (normal oxidation). Marginal deficiencies of thiamin are quite common, usually related to the overconsumption of refined foods, including white flour and sugar, which displace nutrient-rich whole foods in the diet. Symptoms of deficiency include numbness and tingling of the extremities, generalized musculoskeletal tenderness (similar to some of the symptoms of fibromyalgia), heart problems, and a variety of neuropsychological ailments. Low blood pressure and dizziness are also possible signs of inadequate thiamin.

These symptoms have been studied by Dr. Derrick Lonsdale, a preventive medicine physician and researcher, who refers to them as "functional dysautonomia." This refers to abnormalities of the autonomic nervous system, which controls background physiological functions such as temperature, blood pressure, heart rate, glandular secretions, sweating, and intestinal and bladder functions. His research suggests that large doses of thiamin (up to 600 mg daily) may be necessary to correct some of these symptoms.

How to take

Supplements of 50–500 mg are often clinically useful. I usually only suggest 100 mg, the amount that is in the *Basic Multiple,* but on occasion I have suggested more. Another form, much less common but helpful for some people is allithiamin, which is fat soluble.

Niacin and Niacinamide (Vitamin B3)

Niacin is another important B-complex vitamin. It was formerly called nicotinic acid, but the name was changed because it was confused with nicotine by some people. Niacin supplements lower total cholesterol and raise the good (HDL) cholesterol. It was the first nutrient used in the megavitamin treatment of mental disorders, by Drs. Hoffer and Osmond in the early 1950s. The timed-release form of niacin helps to minimize hypoglycemic symptoms, especially during withdrawal from sugar. It usually reduces cravings for sweets. In many patients, high doses help with depression.

Because niacin can dilate blood vessels, it can lower blood pressure and also improve circulation. It can reduce migraine headaches and Raynaud's phenomenon. Many patients who suffer from Meniere's disease, with vertigo or dizzy spells, find relief with niacin supplements. Niacin is one of the nutrients in an orthomolecular program used for the management of drug and alcohol addiction during the withdrawal period.

Plain and sometimes even timed-release niacin can cause a flush of the skin that feels like an allergic reaction. This is secondary to a histamine release, and usually disappears within 15–20 minutes. This flush is usually reduced or eliminated with the timed-release form of niacin, which I have used safely in many patients for years. However, the timed-release niacin can sometimes cause elevation of liver enzymes, and on rare occasions has caused hepatitis in sensitive individuals.

Do not take niacin, either plain or timed release, if you have active peptic ulcer disease or gout (arthritis due to uric acid deposits), since it can increase uric acid levels and gastric acid production. A different form of niacin, inositol hexaniacinate, has several advantages; it causes no flush and has the same cholesterol-lowering capacity as regular niacin. It has never been shown to cause liver problems. The inositol hexaniacinate form does not cause uric acid elevation or histamine-induced gastric acid release and is therefore not a problem in gout or ulcer disease.

How to take

The *Basic Multiple* formula contains 150 mg of niacinamide and 40 mg of niacin (an amount unlikely to cause a flush, although it may in some sensitive people). Niacin is available as 250- to 500-mg timed-release tablets, and inositol hexaniacinate is available as 400-mg capsules. Therapeutic doses of niacin range from 250 mg twice per day up to 1000 mg three times per day. I often suggest 400–800 mg of inositol hexaniacinate twice per day for patients with elevated cholesterol. For hypoglycemics, I often start them on the timed-release form, 250 mg twice per day.

Niacinamide is another form of B3, which does not cause histamine release. It is helpful for osteoarthritis, anxiety, and insomnia, but it does not lower cholesterol levels. The therapeutic doses are generally the same as for niacin. It is often just as beneficial as niacin for certain mental disturbances. For arthritis, the effective dose of niacinamide is between 2 and 3 g to start. These can be reduced to 1000–1500 mg after the symptoms are relieved. It is available as 500-mg capsules or tablets.

Pantothenic Acid (Vitamin B5)

Pantothenic acid was discovered by Dr. Roger Williams, the originator of the concept of biochemical individuality. It is essential for the adrenal glands to produce their hormones. The adrenal glands help maintain us in times of stress, during which they can become severely depleted. They need extra pantothenic acid (as well as vitamin C) to restore normal adrenal function. A deficiency of pantothenic acid can lead to depression, fatigue and insomnia. Requirements for pantothenic acid are higher during pregnancy and lactation. Some physicians are using high doses for arthritis.

I often recommend high doses of pantothenic acid for my patients with recurrent illnesses, environmental toxicity, allergies or high stress levels.

How to take

Pantothenic acid is generally sold as calcium pantothenate, and it is commonly available in 500-mg tablets or capsules, which contain a little bit of calcium in addition to the pantothenate. I usually recommend 500 mg per day as part of *Basic Multiple*. I may suggest up to 2000 mg to those patients experiencing very high stress levels. The coenzyme form, pantethine, is available as a supplement. A daily dose of 900 mg can significantly lower total cholesterol and triglyceride levels, and raise the good HDL-cholesterol levels.

Pyridoxine (Vitamin B6)

Pyridoxine was another discovery of Dr. Albert Szent-Györgyi, in 1938. It is necessary for antibody formation, enzyme activity, smooth muscle function and fatty acid metabolism. It is a cofactor for many enzymes. Deficiencies can lead to anemia and dermatitis. The dermatitis associated with B6 deficiency is easily mistaken for fatty acid deficiency, and it is common for fatty acid deficiency to occur at the same time as increased need for pyridoxine.

Pyridoxine supplements have helped women who have nausea and vomiting of pregnancy and, combined with magnesium, have reduced symptoms of toxemia of pregnancy—this is a condition with fluid retention, high blood pressure, and protein leaking into the urine; if severe it can lead to convulsions. B6 also reduces birth defects. It has been used to treat PMS, depression, childhood autism and asthma. (For asthma, B6 works better when combined with magnesium, vitamin C and some essential fatty acids.)

B6 has also helped to reduce the incidence of the common oxalate type of kidney stones, particularly when taken with magnesium. You can prevent headaches related to MSG in the "Chinese restaurant syndrome" if you take enough B6 in advance. Of course, it is better to avoid the MSG in the first place.

There is a significantly increased risk of heart disease in people with high blood levels of a metabolite called homocysteine. Serum levels of homocysteine may be more significant than cholesterol levels in predicting the risk of heart disease. Your homocysteine level is likely to be increased if you do not have enough B6, B12, folic acid and betaine (derived from choline). Supplements of these nutrients have been shown to reduce homocysteine levels.

Pyridoxine supplements have been helpful in the treatment of peripheral neuropathy (nerve damage to the extremities), but some reports have shown a relationship of very high doses of B6 to the *development* of neuropathy, if taken for many months. The doses that have been harmful were from 2000 to 6000 mg per day, far above the recommended levels for therapeutic supplementation, but it should be used with caution. Isolated reports suggested similar adverse effects with doses as low as 500 mg, but these reports have not been confirmed. Many women have taken this level for treatment of premenstrual syndrome (PMS).

How to take

I usually recommend the 100 mg that is in *Basic Multiple,* but some other multis have reduced the dose of B6 to lower amounts because of the reports of neuropathy. I still think that 100 mg is quite safe. Additional B6 is available as 100-, 250- and 500-mg capsules or tablets. I usually suggest an additional 250 mg for PMS and carpal tunnel syndrome. B6 may lead to intense dreams and restless sleep when taken at night. It is best to take any extra doses with breakfast.

Folic Acid

Folic acid is found largely in "foliage," or green leafy vegetables, from which it gets its name. Also called folate or folacin, this B vitamin is especially important before and during pregnancy. It is necessary for the health of the fetus, preventing the neural tube birth defects, such as spina bifida (incomplete closure of the spine). It has been estimated that 75% of such birth defects could be prevented with folic acid supplements. This information has been known for well over 20 years, but the FDA is only recently allowing such health claims for folic acid. And, even though the birth defect studies were done with supplements, the FDA insists that any label claims on supplements must say it is better to get the folate from food (asking the supplement company to say on their own label that it is better not to take the supplement!). This is simply further evidence of the FDA opposition to supplements.

Folic acid is important in protection from cancer. It is beneficial for reversing cervical dysplasia, which are the precursor cells to cervical cancer seen on abnormal Pap smears. Folic acid is also helpful in preventing lung cancer. It has also been shown to lower blood levels of homocysteine, lowering your risk of heart disease (see pyridoxine).

Folate is also useful for the prevention and treatment of gum disease, the most common cause of tooth loss. It has this protective effect when applied topically to the gums. Unfortunately, folic acid has a reputation for causing vitamin B12 deficiency. This is *not* true. High doses may mask the early signs of B12-deficiency anemia (seen in a microscopic evaluation of the blood), making it somewhat more difficult to detect, but they do not cause it.

With currently available tests for adequacy of B12, the detection of B12-deficiency anemia is not dependent on the blood smear. However, the FDA limitation on the sale of high-dose folic acid remains in effect, ostensibly to protect the consumer. In reality, there is no reason to protect people from something that is harmless.

The maximum over-the-counter dose of folate is 800 mcg (0.8 mg). To get high doses, you have to take multiple pills, or see a physician who can prescribe higher doses. I often recommend doses of 5 mg for women planning pregnancy, or as early in pregnancy as possible. Recent evidence suggests that this same dose will benefit people with osteoarthritis of the hands, and it is very likely that this would also help arthritis of other joints.

Another use of high-dose folic acid is the prevention and treatment of gout. It blocks the activity of xanthine oxidase, an enzyme that leads to the production of uric acid. This is the substance that is deposited in the joints, causing gout, or in the urinary tract, causing kidney stones. For patients with high uric acid, massive doses, up to 80 mg or more, are often helpful. With a comprehensive health program, including a proper diet, doses of 25 mg may be adequate for the treatment of gout.

How to take

In the United States, folic acid is only available in high doses by prescription, but many nutritionally oriented doctors will prescribe it in 5- to 20-mg capsules. If you want to take preventive doses without a doctor, you need to get 800-mcg tablets and take seven per day, for a total daily dose of 5.6 mg. The *Basic Multiple* contains 800 mcg.

Other B Vitamins

There are therapeutic and preventive values for the other substances often considered part of the B complex. Large doses of *para-aminobenzoic acid* (PABA) are helpful in a sclerosing penile disorder called Peyronie's disease.

Dimethyl glycine (DMG) has been called pangamic acid and vitamin B15 in the past, but it is not a true vitamin. It helps to enhance immunity and may improve the utilization of oxygen at the tissue level. It has been shown to enhance endurance in athletes and has been helpful in some cases of autism. I often recommend 125 mg dissolved in the mouth three or four times per day. DMG is an interesting substance in that it is "hygroscopic," meaning it absorbs water from the atmosphere. If left to sit out in the air, it will absorb enough water to dissolve itself. It is therefore packaged in individually wrapped, sealed foil packets.

Choline, a component of lecithin, is manufactured in the body and is a part of the neurotransmitter *acetylcholine*. It has been shown to significantly affect brain function when taken as a supplement. Large doses are helpful in tardive dyskinesia (awkward, uncontrollable, facial and body movements), a condition that results from long-term use of antipsychotic medications called phenothiazines, including Thorazine®, Stelazine®, Mellaril®, Prolixin®, and others.

Inositol is also found in lecithin. Both inositol and choline are important for fatty acid transport, and they have a reputation for lowering cholesterol levels in the blood. However, research shows a number of other dietary supplements to be more effective for lowering cholesterol. Some people find inositol supplements beneficial for anxiety and insomnia.

Choline and inositol are not strictly water soluble, but are more like emulsifiers. Because they have properties of both fat and water solubility, and because of their metabolic properties, they are known as "lipotropic" agents.

How to take

Both choline and inositol are part of compounds known as phospholipids, which are highly concentrated in nervous tissue. Phosphatidyl choline, in granular form, is a concentrate derived from lecithin, with much of the fat removed. Lecithins are found in egg yolks and legumes, especially soybeans. Granular phosphatidyl choline, which is derived from soybeans, contains both choline and inositol, but high amounts are needed for therapeutic levels. Both of these, and phosphatidyl serine, have been thought to be helpful with brain function, particularly memory. However, the high doses needed may cause some digestive upset.

I sometimes recommend 1–2 tbsp of phosphatidyl choline granules per day. There is also a liquid concentrate of phosphatidyl choline that contains a higher concentration of the active ingredients. The amount of choline and inositol in multivitamins is not sufficient for therapeutic purposes.

Glucosamine Sulfate

Glucosamine sulfate is not really a vitamin, but it is the major amino sugar in the body. It is formed from glucose using the amino acid glutamine as the source of the amino group. Amino sugars are important components of connective tissue, including cartilage, the rubbery material in the joints that protects them from wear and tear.

When joints are inflamed from osteoarthritis (degenerative joint disease), supplements of glucosamine sulfate are often helpful in relieving symptoms and restoring joint integrity. Glucosamine sulfate actually stimulates new cartilage formation to protect the bone surface. In fact, studies have shown that taking glucosamine sulfate is better than the usual drugs for arthritis, called nonsteroidal anti-inflammatory drugs (or NSAIDS), like Motrin®, Indocin®, Advil®, and Naprosyn®.

With NSAIDS treatment, the joints are not helped, but the symptoms are frequently relieved—as long as you keep taking the drugs. These drugs have side effects, including ulcers and gastrointestinal bleeding, and beneath the pain relief, the joint destruction continues. Glucosamine sulfate does not have side effects, and after taking it for three to six weeks, it actually reduces symptoms better than the NSAIDS.

How to take

Glucosamine sulfate is usually available as 500-mg capsules, and the usual effective dose is three or four capsules daily. I usually recommend two capsules twice per day. If the situation is more severe, six capsules may be necessary to achieve results. Newly available forms, such as *N*-acetyl glucosamine and glucosamine HCl, have not been proven effective. They are also more expensive, with no apparent advantages over glucosamine sulfate.

Chapter 6

Mineral Supplements

Mineral supplements have a number of health benefits, although the valuable doses are more frequently closer to the RDA than those of other nutrients. Some of the minerals need to be more carefully balanced than the vitamins. There are both major minerals (or macro-minerals), which are those required in larger amounts, and trace minerals (or micro-minerals), which are required in very small daily amounts.

The major minerals are calcium, magnesium, sulfur, potassium, sodium and phosphorus. The trace minerals include chromium, selenium, zinc, manganese, copper, iodine and iron. You do not need to worry about getting too little sodium in the diet. Sodium chloride, or table salt is far too abundant in the American diet, ranging from 5 to 13 g per day, when the need is for a mere ½–1 g per day. Potassium, on the other hand, is sometimes valuable as a supplement, especially if you do not eat a whole-foods diet.

There are also toxic minerals such as lead, mercury, aluminum and cadmium that may interfere with the metabolism and absorption of the nutritional elements. The toxic minerals also have other harmful effects, and some may increase free-radical production. There are only a few minerals that I recommend in amounts greater than the quantity in a good multivitamin/mineral combination such as the formula listed in Chapter 3 (*Basic Multiple*).

Calcium

Calcium is probably the best-known mineral, due to all the publicity given to it by the dairy industry. In fact, you do not need dairy products at all to have adequate dietary calcium (after all, cows don't drink milk!). The need for calcium would probably be much lower than is publicized, if it weren't for the typical poor health habits in developed countries.

Too much sugar, caffeine, alcohol, meat, protein and phosphate-containing sodas all contribute to the apparently higher need for calcium. They either decrease absorption of calcium or increase its excretion. Apparent requirements for calcium are much lower in many less-developed countries, where such inhibiting factors are less common. Absorption of calcium declines with age, and women absorb less than men, regardless of age.

Calcium is the most abundant mineral in the body. Ninety-nine percent of the calcium in the body is found in the bones, where it gives strength to bone tissue. However, the free calcium is also important in many metabolic functions, including muscle contraction, nerve impulses, some hormone regulation and blood clotting. Some studies show a lower incidence of bowel cancer in people who take calcium supplements, and it may help prevent osteoporosis when combined with a number of other equally important nutrients. There is still controversy about the ideal dose of calcium. Whether women need more to prevent osteoporosis and what is the proper dose for cancer prevention are issues that have not been resolved.

How to take

Absorption of calcium is quite variable, depending on the previously listed factors and on stomach acidity. Many different forms of calcium are available. I believe the 500 mg of calcium (as ascorbate) present in *Basic Multiple* is adequate for most people who follow a healthy diet (not just minor variations of the typical American diet). Calcium supplements are better absorbed when taken with meals. If taken late in the day, it may help you sleep and reduce nighttime leg cramps (especially when balanced with magnesium).

When I want to recommend extra calcium, I usually suggest about 250–750 mg of calcium citrate, which is particularly well absorbed. Other forms of calcium, such as carbonate and lactate are well absorbed for most people. All are relatively inexpensive, but carbonate is least costly.

Magnesium

Magnesium is a major mineral which is frequently ignored in medical circles, but it is extremely important. Recently, the medical community has taken a much greater interest in the therapeutic role of magnesium, especially in heart disease. It helps normal heart and muscle function, neurologic function and normal metabolism of fats, and it reduces arrhythmias of the heart, high blood pressure, anxiety, insomnia, and toxemia of pregnancy. It is also an important component of bone, and it is involved in over 300 enzyme systems.

Magnesium is an important part of the treatment of premenstrual syndrome and menstrual cramps. It is commonly low in the diet and in body tissues. I was surprised when I first learned about nutrition (years after medical school) to reread this fact about magnesium in my medical school biochemistry text. It was never taught to me in school. The official requirements for magnesium are 280 mg and 350 mg per day for women and men, respectively. I believe that a healthier recommendation is closer to 500–1000 mg per day and even more for people with heart or neurological problems.

Diuretic drugs cause loss of magnesium in the urine (in addition to the better publicized loss of potassium). Magnesium is also wasted by consumption of caffeine, alcohol and sugar. Low levels are related to fatigue (including chronic fatigue syndrome), allergies, nervousness and irritability, and hyperactivity and bedwetting in children. It is available in a variety of compounds, and they vary in absorption.

When patients are first starting therapy for muscle spasms, acute pain, acute asthma attacks or anxiety, I often treat them with intravenous magnesium supplements (combined with vitamin C and B complex). It is safer, cheaper and more effective than many of the drugs used for these same purposes. This treatment is not well known among physicians, perhaps because it is too inexpensive to be publicized by drug companies.

How to take

I usually recommend taking 500–1000 mg of magnesium each day. *Basic Multiple* contains 500 mg of magnesium, and in addition I might recommend 100–200 mg twice per day as magnesium aspartate, which is well absorbed. For heart patients or asthma patients, I will sometimes recommend even more (up to 1500 mg). High doses may cause some loosening of the bowels, but magnesium has no other side effects unless abused in extremely high doses (for example, by taking antacids in large amounts).

Dolomite is one source of calcium and magnesium. If your digestion is good, it may be well absorbed. In the past some dolomite supplements were contaminated with heavy metals such as lead, but this is not a recent problem. The ratio of calcium to magnesium (2:1) was thought to be ideal at one time, but many of my colleagues now believe that an equal amount (or even more magnesium) is better.

84

Zinc

Zinc is a trace mineral necessary for normal growth and development, and sexual maturation. It is also a cofactor for many enzymes. A large concentration of zinc is found in the skin, nails, retina and testes. It is also a component of a special antioxidant enzyme called *superoxide dismutase* (SOD) that is manufactured in the body. (This enzyme is also dependent on copper and manganese.) SOD is an important oxygen-free-radical scavenger. Zinc and copper need to be taken in balance, since they compete with each other for absorption. There are different opinions on just what a healthy balance is, but a ratio of about 10 to one (zinc to copper) is reasonable.

Supplements of zinc help with burn and wound healing, enhancement of immune function, and the treatment of acne and other skin disorders. It is one of several nutrients helpful in *macular degeneration* (loss of vision in the most sensitive area of the retina).

Zinc is a very important nutrient for mental health and is sometimes useful in the treatment of anorexia, schizophrenia and autism. (For these patients I also suggest supplements of magnesium, niacin, pyridoxine and essential fatty acids). It has recently been reported in the *Journal of the American Medical Association* that supplementing the diet with zinc during pregnancy (25 mg per day) has resulted in larger, healthier babies. This amount is commonly present in prenatal vitamins and other supplements.

Zinc has been used therapeutically in very high doses (up to 150 mg per day) for prostate enlargement, but such doses may not be necessary if you combine this treatment with essential fatty acids, herbs, and other nutrients. With high doses of zinc, special attention has to be paid to the proper mineral balance in the body, especially copper. These doses may decrease the level of good cholesterol (HDL).

Zinc may be helpful in the removal of lead and cadmium from tissues.

How to take

The usual doses that I recommend are in the form of zinc gluconate, which is well absorbed. *Basic Multiple* contains 30 mg of zinc (along with 3 mg of copper for proper balance). I may use an additional 50–100 mg per day for specific conditions. Patients receiving chelation therapy (an intravenous therapy for vascular disease and heavy metal excess) need extra zinc (50–100 mg daily) because so much is excreted in the urine as a result of the treatment.

Zinc gluconate supplements are commonly available in 15- to 50-mg tablets. Although there are data showing some enhanced absorption from *zinc picolinate,* the actual clinical effects are apparently just as good with the less expensive forms, such as zinc gluconate. *Chelated zinc* is another relatively expensive form that is apparently no better clinically.

Selenium

Selenium is a required trace mineral that is important in the fight against excess exposure to free radicals. Adequate intake is associated with a decreased risk of cancer, including colon and breast cancer, and it reduces the incidence of heart disease. Selenium also helps to displace mercury, a toxic heavy metal, from the tissues. Tuna and swordfish, which may have high levels of mercury, also usually have high levels of selenium to balance it. Low levels of selenium lead to seborrheic dermatitis and dandruff. Selenium is another of the nutrients helpful with macular degeneration.

Many people have a low intake of selenium, especially in those geographical areas where the soil selenium has been depleted as a result of ice-age glacial activity. In these areas, the incidence of cancers is higher. Critics of selenium supplementation have said that even though we live in areas with low soil selenium, the food supply comes from all over the country and the world, so local conditions should not make any difference. They have not adequately answered the epidemiological data, which shows that the local amount of selenium in the soil does make a difference in the disease rate.

Selenium is a component of an important antioxidant enzyme—glutathione peroxidase. This is essential for the full activity of vitamin E, because it helps to regenerate the unoxidized form of the vitamin. Deficiency of selenium may also lead to low thyroid function because it is necessary for an enzyme that converts one form of the hormone (thyroxine or T4) to the active form (T3). Severe deficiency can lead to an inflammation of the heart muscle.

How to take

The *Basic Multiple* formula contains 200 mcg of selenium. I often recommend an additional 200–400 mcg per day for patients at high risk of cancer or heart disease, or for those people who want a more vigorous free-radical protective program. It is available in 200-mcg tablets. Any of the available forms of supplemental selenium is effective.

Chromium

Chromium is a trace mineral that is essential for the maintenance of normal blood sugar levels and the transport of sugar into the muscle cells for metabolism. It improves the function of insulin (the pancreatic hormone responsible for sugar regulation), which helps diabetics and hypoglycemics (people with fluctuating blood sugar levels, commonly called low blood sugar). Chromium has been shown to lower total cholesterol levels while at the same time raising the HDL (high-density lipoprotein), or good cholesterol. Insulin regulation affects fat metabolism, and it has been claimed that chromium supplements can help weight loss, but there is not adequate evidence for this.

Chromium is a part of the glucose tolerance factor (GTF), a biologically active substance manufactured in the body, which regulates sugar metabolism. GTF is thought to be a combination of chromium with niacin and several amino acids, but the structure of GTF itself has not been clearly characterized. However, it appears that the material that your body produces is more active than synthetic GTF.

How to take

I usually recommend the 200 mcg in *Basic Multiple*, and this is generally enough for most people. Additional chromium supplements are available as GTF-chromium (which is not actual glucose tolerance factor) and as chromium picolinate, both of which are effective. The value of the picolinate compared to the GTF form has been heavily debated by people with a financial interest in one or the other.

It appears that all supplemental forms of chromium are clinically active, with minor metabolic differences. If there are problems with diabetes, high cholesterol or weight control, I will commonly recommend an additional 400–800 mcg per day. I use the GTF-chromium or a combination of GTF with chromium picolinate, available in 200- to 300-mcg capsules. Chromium is also available in 1000-mcg tablets.

Iron

There is more iron in the body than any other trace element. It is mostly present in the red blood cells as a part of hemoglobin, the molecule that carries oxygen. Iron is also necessary for the activity of a number of enzymes. A deficiency of iron causes anemia resulting in fatigue and listlessness. Perhaps because of its other functions, fatigue may be seen without obvious anemia.

Too much iron can stimulate the production of free radicals, so it is important to be cautious with both iron supplements and food sources. Studies in Finland and elsewhere have shown that excess iron accumulation is a strong risk factor for the development of heart disease. It is also associated with increased cancer rates. Much of this excess iron comes from meat in the diet.

I only recommend supplements of iron if there is a demonstrated need for it, based on clinical and laboratory evidence. Because of poor diet, iron deficiency is quite common. There are increased needs for iron during pregnancy, and infants may also need extra iron. Iron is responsible for many poisonings when children find bottles of iron supplements meant for adults. Make sure the bottles have child-proof caps (although these are sometimes the kind only kids can open), and be sure to keep the bottles out of the reach of children.

How to take

Iron supplements are available in many forms. The most common, iron sulfate, cause constipation and digestive upset, and is not the best absorbed. Ferrous fumarate, in a timed-release, 50-mg tablet is what I usually recommend. The dose needs to be individualized, usually one to three tablets per day until the deficiency is cured. Iron is best absorbed when taken with vitamin C supplements or foods that are rich in vitamin C, such as oranges.

Other Trace Elements

The other trace minerals—copper, manganese, molybdenum, boron, vanadium, cobalt and iodine are also important for health, even though only extremely small amounts are required.

Cobalt is known primarily for its functions related to its presence in vitamin B12, although there is a relationship of non-B12 cobalt to certain enzyme functions.

Manganese is essential for bone and cartilage formation and for the function of one form of the antioxidant enzyme SOD (superoxide dismutase), which protects the mitochondrial membranes (those little intracellular engines again) from oxidation. It is also a cofactor for a number of other enzymes, and it is yet another nutrient helpful with macular degeneration.

Boron, in a dose of 3 mg per day, has been shown to help retain bone density in menopausal women, perhaps because it can increase serum levels of estrogen. Since this information was published, the daily 3-mg dose of boron is now found more often in multivitamin preparations.

Copper is another mineral essential for SOD activity as well as connective tissue maintenance and immune function. Low copper levels can lead to high blood cholesterol. Excess copper has been considered a problem with mental illness, elevated blood pressure and irritability, but many clinicians now feel that too little copper is a more common problem than too much.

The amounts of these trace minerals in the *Basic Multiple* are generally sufficient for most health programs. Sometimes people do need extra copper or manganese, and diabetics may benefit from supplements of vanadium, in the form of vanadyl sulfate. If your multi does not have one of these, they are available as separate supplements.

Iodine is the critical element in thyroid gland hormone, and it also has some special therapeutic uses. It is used medically to treat goiter (swelling of the thyroid with low thyroid function) if the goiter is the result of low iodine intake, which is very rare in this country. It is advisable that iodine supplements be administered by a knowledgeable health practitioner.

There are some other essential trace elements about which less is known, such as silicon, tin, germanium and nickel, and they are not generally included in supplements. They are not specifically added to the *Basic Multiple* formula, nor are they a part of most formulas on the market.

Chapter 7

Dietary Fats and Essential Fatty Acids

Only recently have we developed an understanding of the role of dietary fats in health. Fats are a source of energy (or calories—too many in most cases) and provide structural protection around organs. As we'll see, they are also important components of cell membranes and precursors of important regulatory molecules.

Types of Fats

There are different kinds of fats, including animal fats, vegetable fats, saturated and unsaturated fats, liquid fats (oils) and solid fats. Some saturated fats have been artificially *hydrogenated*. This refers to the addition of hydrogen atoms to carbon atoms that are linked in a chain.

Fats that occur naturally as saturated fats and those that are artificially hydrogenated are solid at room temperature. The artificially saturated fats contain damaging substances called *trans* fats, which do not occur naturally. More about them later. Both animal fat and partially hydrogenated oils can increase inflammation and elevate the amount of cholesterol and fat in the blood. Vegetarian diets generally contain very little saturated fat, although coconut oil and palm oil are vegetarian sources of saturated fat, and some vegetarians do eat dairy products or eggs. *(Vegans* are strict vegetarians who eat no animal products.)

Essential Fatty Acids

Some unsaturated fats are required in the diet and are therefore called *essential fatty acids* or EFAs. These fats are essential for many reasons. They are an important component of cell membranes. These membranes allow passage of molecules in and out of cells and maintain receptors for hormones. Fats are also the building blocks for hormones. EFAs may also be converted into derivatives called *prostaglandins*, important hormone-like regulatory substances.

Good health is also dependent on a proper balance of the different types of fats. *Linoleic* acid is an *omega-6* unsaturated fat, with its first double bond at the sixth position along the carbon chain. It is found in corn and beans. Linoleic acid is converted through a series of steps to a regulatory substance called *prostaglandin E_1*. Prostaglandins regulate many metabolic functions. Minute amounts can cause significant changes in blood pressure, blood clotting, cholesterol levels, inflammatory responses, allergies, hormone activity, immune function, neurologic function and more. Prostaglandin E_1 decreases the tendency of platelets to clump together, decreases inflammation, stabilizes blood sugar and decreases cholesterol. It decreases spasms in arterial and other involuntary muscle.

A deficiency of omega-6 EFA may result in eczema, premenstrual syndrome, breast pain and lumpiness, inflammation and autoimmune problems, hyperactivity in children and hypertension. Many people have adequate intake of these oils but inefficient conversion to the active prostaglandins. Specifically, individuals with a history of allergy, high cholesterol, diabetes, high alcohol intake, trans fat intake, chemical exposures, or specific nutrient deficiencies (particularly of magnesium and vitamin B6) may have difficulty with conversion. In these cases the metabolic block can be bypassed by taking supplements of GLA (*gamma-linolenic* acid), which helps the problems listed above.

The other EFA is called *alpha-linolenic* acid, which is an *omega-3* oil. This oil is even more unsaturated (has more double bonds), with the first double bond at the third position in the carbon chain. This molecular structure gives the oil different properties. Omega-3 oils predominate in fish oils, flax seeds (linseeds) and some nuts, particularly walnuts. Omega-3 oils play a significant role in reducing the risk of coronary heart disease. Scientists have confirmed that populations with higher fish intake have a lower incidence of heart disease. These oils decrease the tendency of platelets to clump together, a reaction involved in the development of atherosclerosis as well as the precipitation of heart attacks. Omega-3 oils also decrease triglycerides, cholesterol and inflammatory reactions.

There is evidence that a deficiency of omega-3 oils is associated with various skin disorders, arthritis and joint stiffness, prostate problems, irritable bowel syndrome, premenstrual syndrome, depression, phobias and schizophrenia. These oils have a short shelf life, and they are generally removed from our food supply through processing for manufacturers' convenience. Deficiencies are therefore common.

Trans Fatty Acids

Let's get back to *trans* fatty acids. In their natural state, edible oils exist in a specific three-dimensional spatial configuration referred to as *cis*. When oils are highly processed during hydrogenation with heat and catalysts, they are partially converted to a different configuration called *trans*. These fatty acids do not participate in the normal pathways of fatty acid metabolism. They actually block the conversion of the natural cis fats to their active metabolites. *Partially saturated or partly hydrogenated* oil almost invariably contains trans fats. Oils that have been made into margarine contain significant amounts of trans fats, although food processors have made recent efforts to reduce the trans fat content of some margarines. Most processed foods and baked goods contain partially hydrogenated oils, and there is now a significant amount of these abnormal fats in the Western diet. These fats increase the risk of developing heart disease and cancer more than natural saturated fats. In addition, trans fats interfere with normal immune function.

It is important to have the right amount of EFAs in the diet or as supplements. Be sure that you use any oils sparingly, because they also lead to excess caloric intake and weight gain.

The metabolism and clinical use of the essential fatty acids has been one of the remarkable developments in medicine in the past decade. The education of physicians regarding these oils is due in part to the work of two physicians, David Horrobin, MD, and Donald Rudin, MD, who have done research and scoured the literature and reported on the physiology of fats and oils. A recent book, *Fats That Heal, Fats That Kill*, by Udo Erasmus, is a thorough review of fats and oils.

Many open-minded clinicians who have tried these essential fatty acid supplements have been impressed with the results in their patients, and they are now an important component of nutritional therapeutics. On the basis of the research and the teaching of these doctors, I tried these treatments in my practice and found them to be beneficial for a variety of clinical problems. They are safe, easy to take, and relatively inexpensive.

Essential Fatty Acid Supplements

EPA

EPA stands for eicosapentaenoic acid, so it is obvious why we call it simply EPA. This is a fish oil concentrate that is rich in omega-3 oil that has already started its conversion to prostaglandin E_3. Fish oils also contain DHA (docosahexaenoic acid), another omega-3 essential fatty acid, which has similar properties.

Fish oil supplements have been shown to reduce inflammation, especially in arthritis, and to reduce rejection reactions after organ transplants, without the side effects of some of the anti-rejection drugs. They also lower cholesterol levels and reduce platelet stickiness. This reduces the risk of clots inside the blood vessels. They can help with some of the symptoms of premenstrual syndrome, bowel dysfunction and mental illness. Fish oil supplements can lower cholesterol levels in the blood, help to lower blood pressure, and reduce excessive blood clotting (platelet activity). It is helpful in heart and blood vessel disease.

How to take

The usual therapeutic dose of fish oils ranges from 3 to 12 g per day. Capsules of 1000 mg (containing 180 mg of EPA and 120 mg of DHA) are commonly available, and there are also some supplements with a higher concentration of the active oils. Sometimes higher doses are used in studies, but with comprehensive diet and supplement programs it is usually possible to achieve beneficial effects with lower doses. I usually recommend starting on two to four capsules per day, and may increase the dose if the response is not adequate.

Flax Seed Oil

Another good source of omega-3 oil is flax seeds. Many of the effects are similar to fish oil, but because they have not yet gone through the first step in conversion they may not be as helpful in some situations. Supplements of flax seed oil are useful in a variety of skin disorders, including psoriasis, and digestive problems, including spastic colon and probably inflammatory bowel disease. Some claims have been made for benefits in other inflammatory diseases, as well as cancer and immune system problems.

How to take

Usual doses of flax seed oil are 1–3 tbsp per day for therapeutic purposes, reducing this to 1–3 tsp after the desired effect is achieved. It is available in 8.8- and 17.6-ounce bottles. It is important that the processing of the oil is done in an inert gas environment and that the oil is stored in opaque bottles without oxygen. This oil is very easily oxidized especially if exposed to heat and light, and I recommend keeping it in the freezer until it is opened, and then in the refrigerator. (After taking it out of the freezer it will take a few minutes to liquefy.) It is a good idea never to cook with flax oil because of its sensitivity to heat, but you may safely add it to hot foods after cooking.

Flax seeds themselves are a good source of the omega-3 oil and a large amount of fiber, especially soluble fiber. Each tablespoon of seeds contains about one teaspoon of oil. The fiber in flax seeds is an effective treatment for both constipation and diarrhea, and it helps to eliminate toxins. Grinding the seeds only for immediate use (in a small electric coffee mill) provides the freshest source of the oil. I like to grind up some flax seeds and add them to a blender drink with banana, other fruit, dilute juice and low-fat organic yogurt.

Gamma-Linolenic Acid (GLA)

Gamma-linolenic acid, or GLA, is found in evening primrose oil, borage oil and black currant oil. GLA is produced by enzyme action on the linoleic acid that is essential in the diet. It is the result of the first step in conversion to the beneficial prostaglandin PGE_1, bypassing the metabolic blockages mentioned above. Supplements have anti-inflammatory effects because they lead to increased production of the PGE_1.

Many studies have shown remarkable benefits from supplements of GLA. It helps relieve premenstrual symptoms, asthma and eczema and other autoimmune disorders. It can lower blood pressure in hypertension and decrease excessive blood clotting. It helps to regulate hormonal function through its effect on production and release of hormones and through control of hormone activity at the target organs. GLA has been shown to help in alcoholism, diabetes, acne, hyperactivity and numerous other conditions. Although it sounds miraculous, its effects are easily explainable based on well-known nutritional biochemistry.

How to take

I usually recommend the borage oil source of GLA, since it is the most cost effective and concentrated, meaning that fewer pills are necessary. It comes in 1000-mg capsules, which contain 240 mg of GLA. One per day is usually adequate. Evening primrose oil contains 40 mg of GLA per 500-mg capsule (usual dose—six per day); and black currant oil contains about 80 mg per capsule, and three per day is an adequate dose. After therapeutic results, the dose may be lowered for maintenance.

Chapter 8

Amino Acid Supplements

Amino acids are the building blocks of protein molecules. They are also components of neurotransmitters, nitrogen sources for nucleic acids (DNA and RNA), and the foundation of certain hormones (insulin, for example). Enzymes are made up of protein molecules. Several of the amino acids are therapeutically useful. Some amino acids are essential (required in the diet). Some of them are produced in the body but in less-than-ideal amounts. In these situations, supplements are extremely valuable. Also, in certain health problems the need for amino acids rises dramatically.

FDA Bans Tryptophan

In 1989 the United States Food and Drug Administration (FDA) removed a very valuable amino acid—tryptophan—from the supplement market because of a single contaminated batch that was imported from a single manufacturer in Japan. The contaminant was soon revealed to be the result of a new manufacturing process, and the problem was solved. This information was published in the *New England Journal of Medicine* and the *Journal of the American*

Medical Association as well as toxicology journals, but as of this writing the FDA has not yet returned tryptophan to the dietary supplement market.

There is only one possible (although unacceptable) explanation for this—politics. Tryptophan is a safe and inexpensive competitor to a drug, and the FDA has a long history of opposition to the therapeutic value of nutrients. Uncontaminated tryptophan is safe *even by the FDA's own standards*, since it is approved by the FDA for use in infant formulas, total intravenous feeding formulas, and in animal feed. The FDA position is being challenged, and I anticipate dramatic changes in their unduly harsh regulations, without any sacrifice of public safety. (See Chapter 13.)

Because amino acids are present in large amounts in food, it is common for supplements to be more effective when taken separate from meals containing other protein sources. Since they are not given for their protein value as much as for their precursor value, they may be "drowned out" by other amino acids from typical high-protein foods. Unfortunately, people frequently forget to take supplements separately from mealtimes, so you are more likely to take amino acid supplements successfully if you do so with your meals. Taking at least some of the dose at bedtime and on arising is a reasonable alternative and may be easier to remember. Dietary supplements that you do not remember to take are 100% ineffective.

Amino Acids and Proteins

In the United States and other developed countries, many people actually consume too much protein, although not necessarily in the right balance. Too much protein creates a nitrogen overload on the liver and kidneys, and people with liver or kidney disorders must be extremely cautious about consuming any extra amino acids. If you take therapeutic levels of amino acids, it is usually a good idea to reduce other protein sources (unless you are already on a low-protein vegetarian diet). Amino acid names are usually preceded by the letter "L" referring to their ability to rotate the plane of polarized light in a "left-handed" direction. This is the usual natural form of the molecule. The letter may be left out in the text. (The "D" form is normally only used as a supplement in the DL-form of phenylalanine.)

L-*Glutamine*

L-Glutamine is the most abundant free amino acid in the bloodstream. It helps build muscle, especially in times of stress or illness. It is an important transporter of nitrogen. It is an important energy source for the intestinal lining cells, and it is essential for immune function. Glutamine is critically important in the healing of peptic ulcers and inflammatory bowel disease and in treating diarrhea. Supplements of glutamine may dramatically improve recovery after surgery or trauma and it can hasten the healing of wounds.

L-Glutamine reduces cravings due to low blood sugar and also helps to improve memory. The brain usually burns sugar (glucose) as its main fuel. When sugar levels are low, neurologic and psychiatric symptoms can develop. However, the brain can use glutamine as an alternative fuel to decrease those mental symptoms. It can reduce depression and fatigue. Glutamine is also an important antioxidant precursor, since the body uses it to make glutathione, an antioxidant enzyme.

How to take

Glutamine supplements are readily available in 500-mg capsules, and it is also available as a pure powder that can be mixed with water or dilute juice when very high doses are needed. (When looking for supplements, be sure to specify glutamine, not glutamate or glutamic acid.) I will frequently recommend two or three capsules twice per day (2000–3000 mg total), and sometimes up to 4500 mg per day. Higher doses of glutamine are useful for more severe inflammatory bowel conditions, wasting diseases, and ulcers. Researchers are still evaluating the use of high doses of glutamine for immune function disorders such as AIDS, but the preliminary results are very promising.

L-*Carnitine*

L-Carnitine is an amino acid necessary for the metabolism of fat in the cells. Fat is burned for energy in cells by the mitochondria. The mitochondria are surrounded by a membrane, and carnitine is essential for the passage of fat across this membrane. As a consequence, carnitine enhances the burning of fat, lowers the triglyceride (fat) level in the blood, and may make it easier for some people to lose weight.

Your body makes carnitine from other amino acids (lysine and methionine), so it is not considered essential, but the production is often low, especially in disease states. L-Carnitine levels are high in muscle, especially heart muscle, but it is very low in that of patients with arteriosclerosis (hardening of the arteries). It improves the skeletal and heart muscle energy.

Larger doses of L-carnitine (1000–2000 mg per day) are effective for the relief of angina pectoris (heart pain due to diminished oxygen), but it is especially valuable if given for a period of time before symptoms occur. In allowing more burning of fat, it reduces the muscle dependency on glucose. When glucose is burned with too little oxygen (as in hardening of the arteries or intense muscle activity), the extra lactic acid produced leads to increased pain (as in a racer's calf muscles). For the same reason, it can improve energy, stamina and recovery rate in athletes.

How to take

I usually recommend capsules of 250 mg, and suggest taking two or three capsules twice per day. Much higher levels have been given experimentally with no side effects, and they appear to be helpful in some cases. Carnitine is quite safe. Although I usually take only a moderate amount of L-carnitine, on occasion I have taken as much as 5 g (20 capsules) in one day, as an experiment to increase athletic stamina. There were no side effects, but neither did I notice any special results. (Since I usually feel good, it is difficult to draw conclusions without doing scientific studies. Fortunately, such studies have been done, and they do show the value of carnitine for increasing stamina.)

Phenylalanine

Phenylalanine is an essential amino acid that, in addition to its role in protein formation, is a precursor of several important metabolites. It can be made into another amino acid called tyrosine, and from there into the adrenal hormones, including *norepinephrine*. Norepinephrine (structurally similar to adrenaline) is a neurotransmitter. Tyrosine is also metabolized into melanin, the skin pigment. Metabolic addition of iodine to tyrosine leads to the formation of thyroid hormone.

Unlike most amino acids, phenylalanine has therapeutic value in two forms. DL-Phenylalanine (DLPA) is used in the treatment of chronic pain syndromes. L-Phenylalanine (LPA) is used for the treatment of depression. LPA differs from tryptophan in its effect on depression, because it is a precursor of a different neurotransmitter.

How to take

Both L-phenylalanine and DL-phenylalanine are commonly available as 500-mg capsules, and I frequently recommend 1000–2000 mg of LPA twice per day for depression. I suggest taking at least part of the dose at bedtime. For chronic pain, DLPA is often effective at 500 mg, taken several times per day.

L-Arginine

L-Arginine is a nonessential amino acid that is a precursor of nitric oxide. Nitric oxide is an arterial wall muscle relaxant (known as *endothelial-derived relaxing factor)* that helps to open up the arteries. As a consequence, arginine supplements may help with hypertension and coronary artery disease. Nitroglycerin is useful for the treatment of angina pectoris (chest pain from coronary artery disease) because it releases nitric oxide.

Arginine has also been shown to reduce chemical carcinogenesis (production of cancer). It has been touted as a muscle builder because of its potential to stimulate the release of growth hormone from the pituitary gland, but this has not been clearly shown to happen in humans who take arginine supplements. Some reports suggest that the balance of arginine and lysine (another amino acid) is important in recurrence rates of infections with *Herpes simplex* virus. Too much arginine may precipitate outbreaks of herpes, and thus it must sometimes be balanced with supplements of lysine.

Arginine can enhance hormone release, improve immunity and increase the rate of wound healing after trauma, burns or surgery. It may be of help in asthma because the nitric oxide it produces is also a relaxant of the bronchial (airway) muscles.

How to take

I have used 500–1000 mg of arginine twice per day, but higher doses may help some conditions. Some people are taking up to 6 g per day. Arginine is commonly available in 500-mg capsules and is also available as a powder to make it easier to take higher doses.

L-Lysine

L-Lysine is an essential amino acid. It is therapeutic for the treatment of herpes, especially when combined with relatively low arginine intake. It has been suggested that high doses of lysine may stimulate increased production of cholesterol by the liver, but in my experience this is not very common. On the other hand, lysine is a precursor of carnitine, and carnitine helps to lower triglyceride and cholesterol levels. There is some evidence that lysine supplements can help with the treatment of heart and blood vessel disease (atherosclerosis).

How to take

The usual dose of lysine for prevention of herpes is 500–1000 mg per day. When an outbreak occurs, the dose may be increased to 2000–4000 mg per day. With this dose, the lesions heal faster and the recurrences are less frequent. It comes in 500-mg capsules.

L-Taurine

L-Taurine is one of the few sulfur-containing amino acids (others are cysteine and methionine). Although it is not essential, because it can be made from cysteine, it is not always made in adequate amounts for optimal physiological function. Sulfur carriers are important antioxidants. Taurine is important for solubility of the bile and may help prevent or treat gallstones. It is also involved in stabilizing cell membranes, and it therefore affects nerve conduction and hypersensitivity.

Taurine has a role in balancing sodium and potassium in the heart muscle and other cells, and it helps increase the strength of the heartbeat in congestive heart failure. In some fad liquid-protein diets of the late 1970s and early 1980s, serious complications resulted because they contained inadequate taurine. This prevented proper uptake of potassium into the heart muscle, leading to arrhythmias. Clinical experience shows that taurine is helpful for patients with various heart rhythm problems (skipped beats or palpitations). It also helps to lower blood pressure if it is abnormally high.

Taurine is concentrated in the retina of the eye, where it is concentrated in the cells that receive light, and it is likely to be helpful in treating and preventing age-related macular degeneration. It also helps prevent damage from ultraviolet light and some toxic substances.

How to take

Taurine is available as 500-mg capsules, and I usually recommend one or two of these twice per day for heart failure or arrhythmia patients. The same amount has been helpful for some seizure disorders. For preventing eye disorders, one or two capsules may be adequate (although sometimes it is given intravenously in higher doses).

In reviewing the research, you will find that up to 12 capsules per day have been used in heart disease studies. However, these doses may not be needed when taurine is used in combination with other nutrients. This is a common finding in clinical practice, as compared with research in which a substance is used alone for clearer results.

L-*Tryptophan*

L-Tryptophan is an essential amino acid which is an important precursor to both serotonin and melatonin. As a precursor of serotonin, a neurotransmitter, it has profound effects on brain function. Increasing brain levels of serotonin with supplements of tryptophan have relieved both depression and insomnia.

Some of the most popular recent drug prescriptions for depression (Prozac®, Zoloft®) are effective specifically because they result in increased levels of serotonin in the brain. Some people have speculated that the reason the FDA removed tryptophan from the market had more to do with its competition with drugs than with the isolated, temporary contamination problem.

Although tryptophan is not currently available as an over-the-counter supplement for human consumption as of this writing (1995), the common dosage form that was available before the FDA ban was capsules of 500 mg. I have recommended doses of 1000–4000 mg per day, usually starting with 1000 mg twice per day, including one dose at bedtime. Unfortunately, many patients who depended on tryptophan to keep them in good mental health, or for restorative sleep, have been forced either to suffer or to take medications. These drugs frequently have side effects not seen with tryptophan. It is my honest hope that tryptophan will soon be back on the market. It is currently available as a prescription in Canada, and some people are purchasing it legally for "veterinary use" in the United States.

Melatonin

Melatonin is not an amino acid, but it is a hormone that is manufactured in the pineal gland from the amino acid tryptophan. The pineal gland is a pea-sized organ that sits at the base of the brain. Melatonin is also available as a dietary supplement. It is the substance that appears to regulate the "body clock," the physiological changes that relate to day-night changes.

Melatonin levels normally go up when it turns dark, and they are low during daylight hours. This hormone is also an antioxidant/free-radical scavenger that appears to slow the aging process. The production of melatonin is high in youth and declines steadily with age. Many signs of aging are associated with this loss of melatonin production, but cause and effect have not been proven. Large doses of melatonin have been administered to animals and humans without any known side effects.

Supplements of melatonin, taken at night, often help with insomnia and in overcoming symptoms of jet lag (for jet lag, it is taken near the bedtime in the new time zone for two or three days before departure and after arrival). Unlike most medications for insomnia, melatonin is not addictive. When it is used for insomnia, it does not leave you with any hangover or withdrawal symptoms. Some animal and human studies have shown benefits in reducing cancer and enhancing immune function. In animal studies, there is a clear increase in longevity (unfortunately, it is difficult to do longevity studies in humans). In humans, it has helped in treating depression and also in lowering the eye pressures in patients with glaucoma.

How to take

Melatonin is commonly available in 3-mg capsules or tablets, and the usual dose is 3–6 mg at bedtime. Sometimes higher doses are helpful for insomnia and depression. Some people seem to benefit from taking 10–15 mg of melatonin, without developing any apparent side effects. Larger doses are being studied for birth control because of melatonin's effect on sexual hormone balance.

Supplements of melatonin are almost all synthetically produced, but the synthetic molecules are identical to the natural human melatonin. There may be some brands on the market that contain actual animal pineal gland, but I do not recommend these. They are not as well standardized and they may contain impurities. Synthetic melatonin supplements are pure white, while the gland sources usually have some coloration.

Chapter 9

Flavonoids, Herbs
and Botanicals

Flavonoids

There is a wide variety of *phytochemicals* (plant chemicals) that have physiological functions. Some of the newer
ones have had a lot of press in the mid-1990s as a result of
their role in protecting against cancer and heart disease, as
well as many other illnesses. (Of course, all vitamins are
also phytochemicals, and well-known herbs also contain
them, they are just not as newsworthy, as far as the press is
concerned.)

The flavonoids (also called bioflavonoids) are phytochemical pigments that act as antioxidants to protect plants
(and the animals that eat these plants, including you) from
excess oxygen/free-radical damage. They enhance vitamin
C activity and improve the strength of blood vessels, thus
reducing bruising, bleeding gums and the development of
varicose veins and hemorrhoids. They have a host of other
physiological effects.

Various flavonoids also help prevent cataract progres-
sion and macular degeneration, and they have been used to
treat menopausal hot flashes. Bioflavonoids are also potent

anti-inflammatory, anti-allergic, anticancer and antiviral agents. Some of the most recently available dietary supplements, such as quercetin, ginkgo extract, proanthocyanidins, and bilberry, contain substances in the bioflavonoid family. Lutein is a flavonoid that has recently become available as a supplement and helps prevent macular degeneration. Some of the flavonoids are not yet available as supplements, once again calling attention to the importance of eating a healthy, whole-foods diet.

Genistein is an "isoflavonoid," found in soy products, that decreases the spread of tumors. It prevents the development of new blood vessels, reducing the supply of oxygen and nourishment to the tumor cells. Genistein also acts as a weak estrogen, blocking stronger estrogens from attaching to their receptor sites and preventing the stimulation which may give rise to cancer. Cultures with high soy intake have lower rates of breast and prostate cancers. Soy milk, tofu, tempeh and miso are all good sources of genistein. As of this writing, it is not available as a supplement, but since soy products are versatile and readily available, there is no real need for a supplement.

Herbs/Botanicals

In addition to those that contain flavonoids, there are many plant-derived health products that come from many cultural heritages and healing arts throughout the ages. Many of our modern drugs were derived originally from herbal remedies. Digitalis, used in treating some heart diseases, comes from foxglove. Colchicine, a common treatment for gout, comes from colchicum, or autumn crocus. Some of the more potent medications for cancer come from common vinca plants.

Most of the common herbs used in health care are very safe when used as directed, and far safer than almost any prescription medication, but it is valuable to have competent advice when using them for treatment, even if only for a proper diagnosis of the problem. Many certified nutritionists know how to use herbs in health care. There are some physicians who are knowledgeable about botanical remedies. For the most part they are naturopathic physicians, or NDs (Doctors of Naturopathy), but many chiropractors and some MDs who have sought special training know quite a lot about this field.

There are many treatises on herbs in health care, but this is not one of them. I do use a number of herbal preparations in practice, and information on these is worth reporting. Most of the time they are used for treatment of specific conditions, but some of them are used for general toning and prevention. For more thorough discussions of herbal remedies, see the books listed in the Resources section. (See Appendix 2.)

Herbs are not orthomolecular substances. Unlike nutrients, they contain components that are not normally present in the body. Although they are used for treatment and general toning, be aware that they are more likely than nutrients to have side effects when taken in high doses. The usual doses are quite safe, but you should not exceed them unless you are familiar with their use.

Mixed Bioflavonoids

There are many available supplements of 500–1000 mg of mixed bioflavonoids, usually consisting of hesperidin, rutin and citrus extracts. At one time the flavonoids were referred to as vitamin P, a term introduced by Albert Szent-Györgyi. I often recommend a supplement tablet containing 1000 mg of mixed flavonoids, once or twice per day, for their general antioxidant activity, enhancement of blood vessel strength, support for the actions of vitamin C, and to treat hot flashes associated with menopause. Citrus bioflavonoids have been shown to protect tissues from the effects of radiation.

Sometimes bioflavonoids are mixed with vitamin C and the combination is referred to as vitamin C complex. However, it is usually less expensive and more flexible to take vitamin C and the bioflavonoids separately—you can then vary the doses independently. Other specific bioflavonoids have general antioxidant benefits and some more specific effects.

Quercetin

This brilliant yellow-green bioflavonoid has a special effect on certain cell membranes. It has an affinity for the cells that release histamine and serotonin, the mediators of the allergic and inflammatory responses. It stabilizes the membranes of these *mast cells* and *basophils*, reducing their chemical release. These membranes are often leaky in allergy sufferers, allowing excessive release of the allergy mediators. It can also help asthma patients, reducing their sensitivity to allergens. Interestingly, a drug with a similar effect, cromolyn, is a synthetic flavonoid.

Quercetin reduces the activity of an enzyme called aldose reductase. This in turn decreases the deposition of sugar-protein complexes in the lens of the eye, and lowers your risk of developing cataracts. Limiting sugar intake is also helpful with cataract prevention, especially the milk sugar lactose, because of the effect of one of its components—galactose—on increasing cataract formation. Another effect of quercetin is to reduce the damage induced by tobacco smoke in the airway membranes. Even if you do not smoke yourself, it is hard to completely avoid exposure to secondhand smoke.

How to take

I usually suggest doses of 400 mg of quercetin twice per day for allergic patients and those at risk of cataract. Often, they need to increase the dose to 1200 or 1600 mg per day for asthma or nonresponsive allergy symptoms. The product I use contains 400 mg of quercetin, mixed with the enzyme bromelain to help enhance its absorption.

Ginkgo biloba

Ginkgo biloba extract comes from the leaf of the ancient tree of the same name. The extract contains terpene substances, known as ginkgolides and bilobalides, which improve circulation to the brain in patients with hardening of the arteries. This increases the oxygen supply and availability of other nutrients to the brain and results in generally improved central nervous system function. It has been shown in scientific studies to improve memory, especially short-term memory, to enhance concentration, and to relieve associated depression.

Ginkgo also contains a variety of bioflavonoids that act as free-radical scavengers and antioxidants. In addition to these nonspecific benefits and memory enhancement, ginkgo extract helps with peripheral vascular disease, vertigo (dizziness), tinnitus (ringing in the ears), migraine headaches and Raynaud's phenomenon. Because degenerative eye diseases, such as macular degeneration, are probably related to oxidation and poor microcirculation, ginkgo has been suggested for these conditions.

Most of the scientific studies on *Ginkgo biloba* have been done with a 24% *standardized extract,* not the plain powdered leaf. Capsules of the powdered leaf are also available, but the level of active components is not as consistent as in the standardized product.

How to take

Capsules of the 24% standardized *Ginkgo biloba* extract are available in 40- to 60-mg sizes. I usually recommend taking about 120 mg per day (two or three capsules depending on the size), although I have sometimes recommended higher doses.

Proanthocyanidins

Proanthocyanidin (PAC) bioflavonoids (also called procyanidolic oligomers) are powerful antioxidants and free-radical scavengers. A number of physiological and nutritional substances appear to have difficulty getting into the brain tissue, which has led to the surmise that there is a physiological barrier, not an actual physical wall, protecting the brain. Proanthocyanidins, however, do cross this so-called *blood-brain barrier*, which allows them to act as antioxidants in the brain. The brain is largely made up of fatty tissue that is prone to oxidative damage.

Proanthocyanidins are helpful in slowing the aging process, improving blood vessel and connective tissue strength and detoxifying the body. They often help with allergies and as anti-inflammatory agents. PACs may reduce the risk of cancer, heart disease, and stroke and reduce the inflammation in arthritis.

The PACs are natural plant products, which were first studied as supplements derived from the bark of a European pine tree (the Pycnogenol® brand). These compounds and other related substances are also found in grape seed extracts, which are now available as supplements. Most of the research by the originator, Dr. Jacques Masquelier, has been done with the grape seed extract, which he endorses as the preferred source. It is also cheaper than the pine bark extract.

The latest information is that the grape seed is an even better source of active product, although there are compounds present in each source that are not present in the other. We now know that they act within cell membranes, and they neutralize both water- and fat-soluble free radicals. They also inhibit the release of enzymes that damage capillaries. Proanthocyanidins have been shown to be safe in numerous tests over many years.

How to take

Both grape seed and pine bark extracts are available individually or as mixtures. I usually recommend a 50-mg capsule twice per day of a mixture containing 40 mg of grape seed extract and 10 mg of pine bark extract. Sometimes people start with higher doses and then taper down to 50–100 mg per day.

Garlic

Garlic has a long history of use in culinary arts, but it also has been used as a healing substance for centuries. It has been studied extensively in recent years, and the findings confirm many of its historical uses. Garlic reduces excessive blood clotting by decreasing platelet stickiness (platelets are small disk-shaped structures in the blood that initiate blood clots).

Garlic, as a food or a supplement, lowers cholesterol and blood pressure and helps to kill yeast in the intestinal tract. It contains sulfur compounds (allylic sulfides) that help to detoxify many carcinogens and protect you from developing cancer. They are also being studied in the treatment of cancer. The substances that produce the odor in garlic are excreted by the lungs, leading to "garlic breath." They also come out through the pores of the skin.

There are many different garlic preparations on the market, and they are being highly publicized. The most potent preparations are the "deodorized" forms (not "odorless," which is also sold), which contain the equivalent of many cloves of garlic in each pill. According to researchers, each of the brands that they used in their studies was effective in producing experimental responses.

How to take

Deodorized garlic powder is commonly available in 350- to 500-mg capsules. I usually suggest taking one or two of the 500-mg capsules twice per day. It is also available as a liquid, but this is not as convenient as the capsules. In case you are wondering, the deodorized brands do not leave you with "garlic breath."

Bilberry

Several species of blueberry (as well as other berries and cherries) contain compounds called anthocyanosides (similar to proanthocyanidins), which appear to have antioxidant properties and other therapeutic value.

Bilberry helps enhance vision and adaptation to the dark and improves capillary circulation, which is especially important in the retina. It is also useful for diabetic visual impairment and for improving the health of the macula of the retina, where clearest vision takes place.

Loss of vision is one of the most feared medical conditions. Visual deterioration is so common with advancing age, from cataract, diabetes, hardening of the arteries, and age-related macular degeneration, that it is important to be careful with all health practices that may affect eyesight. Aside from the usual recommendations for diet and exercise, adding bilberry and other specific nutrient supplements is prudent for treatment and prevention.

How to take

I have recommended bilberry extract as part of a comprehensive program for patients who have visual problems. Bilberry extract is available as a single ingredient, in 100-mg tablets or capsules. It is also frequently made as a combination of 100 mg of bilberry with other nutrients that protect the eye. It should say on the label that it is standardized to contain from 15 to 25% anthocyanosides. I usually recommend taking one capsule two or three times per day.

The combination that I use as vision nutrients contains 100 mg of the standardized bilberry extract, plus taurine, trace minerals, proanthocyanidins, *Ginkgo biloba* and other antioxidants. Higher bilberry doses may help cataracts.

Silymarin (Milk Thistle Extract)

Silymarin is a combination of several components extracted from milk thistle. These are flavonoid antioxidants with specific benefits for the liver. They aid in the healing of already damaged liver, and they protect the liver from the damaging effects of environmental chemicals. As with other flavonoids, some of the benefits are the result of reduced cell-membrane damage induced by free radicals. Silymarin also improves sugar levels in diabetics and reduces their urinary sugar spillover. It reduces capillary fragility and excess blood vessel permeability.

Silymarin probably produces some of its clinical effects by restoring liver cell membranes and by increasing the sensitivity of insulin receptors. As a result, diabetics can safely decrease their insulin doses. (Do not do so without medical supervision.) Interestingly, silymarin is used to treat liver diseases in many countries other than the United States. Generally, the US medical profession has been resistant to the use of herbal preparations.

How to take

Supplements of milk thistle extract, standardized with 80% silymarin, are available in 150-mg capsules. Two capsules twice per day is an effective dose for liver protection and sugar improvement. For general protection, one or two capsules per day may be adequate, unless you are highly exposed to damaging environmental chemicals.

Saw Palmetto

The saw palmetto tree (*Serenoa repens*) is a small palm tree that produces reddish-brown berries that are therapeutic for prostate gland enlargement. The prostate gland is the male organ (about the size of a walnut) located under the bladder and surrounding the neck of the bladder and the urine outflow channel—the urethra. Certain fat-soluble substances in the berries (saponins and phytosterols) help to reduce benign enlargement of the prostate, and this relieves abnormal pressure on the urethra.

Benign enlargement of the prostate is very common in men over 40. A recently developed drug may also help the prostate, but it has side effects and it is not as effective as the saw palmetto extract, which is safer. (The FDA sees fit to allow medical claims for the drug, but not health claims for the herbal extract.) *Saw palmetto* is part of a comprehensive approach to the treatment of prostate enlargement.

Symptoms of prostate enlargement are difficulty starting urination, slow urine flow, frequent urination, urgency, retained urine in the bladder, dripping after completion of urination, and nighttime urination interrupting sleep. Saw palmetto extract helps all of these symptoms by interfering with the production of a testosterone metabolite (dihydrotestosterone) that is a strong stimulant to prostate enlargement.

How to take

Saw palmetto is available as 120- to 160-mg capsules. The usual therapeutic level is 300–500 mg per day. I recommend the 160-mg capsules taken twice per day, and an additional capsule if the symptoms are not responding or are particularly severe. The alternative is to take a less effective medication or to wait until the symptoms are severe enough to require surgical reduction of prostate tissue.

I have recently added two other herbs to my treatment of symptomatic prostate enlargement. One of them is *Pygeum africanum,* and the other is *Urtica dioica* (stinging nettle). These appear to reduce the irritation and sensitivity of the bladder and urethra, reducing the symptoms of frequency and urgency. The typical dose is 25 mg of *Pygeum* and 125 mg of stinging nettle, each taken twice per day.

Echinacea

These two herbal species, both *Echinacea angustifolia* and *Echinacea purpurea,* are commonly used for enhancement of the immune system. They contain *echinacosides* and *sesquiterpenes,* which enhance white blood cell activity and increase interferon production. Echinacea increases both the number and activity of the white blood cells known as T-cells and the natural killer cells. As is true of many herbs, very high doses may have side effects. However, the usual doses are generally quite safe.

Echinacea has antiviral and antibacterial activity, and it is useful in treating infections, although with serious bacterial infections I would also recommend the appropriate antibiotic. Echinacea has helped reduce the growth of herpesviruses, which cause genital herpes and cold sores (fever blisters). Because it stimulates white blood cells, echinacea may be helpful in supporting cancer treatments.

How to take

Echinacea is available as capsules or tinctures, but the capsules are usually more convenient. Some people prefer the herbal tinctures diluted in water. Standardized echinacea capsules are available, and I now recommend a mixture containing 125 mg each of the angustifolia and purpurea varieties.

Licorice Extract (DGL)

This is an extract of licorice that has had the *glycyrrhizin* removed. Glycyrrhizin is a component of licorice with some possible toxicity, although it has antiviral activity and some other therapeutic uses. At high doses, the glycyrrhizin may cause elevation of blood pressure due to its hormone-like effects.

The deglycyrrhizinated licorice (you can see why it is called DGL) is activated when chewed well and mixed with saliva. It then coats the esophagus and stomach, forming a protective layer against stomach acid. It can relieve the symptoms of hiatal hernia, gastritis and ulcer, thus letting the tissues heal, without the need for antacids or antihistamine drugs such as Zantac®. Comparative studies show that DGL is as good as the antihistamine drugs for the treatment of stomach and duodenal ulcers.

The real problem with peptic ulcers is not usually too much acid in the stomach, but rather an increased sensitivity of the lining cells to normal levels of acid. There is also reason to suspect that a refined food diet, with low fiber and lots of sugar, plus coffee consumption contribute to the causation of ulcer disease, along with high stress levels.

Current information shows that there is a bacterium, called *Helicobacter pylori*, which causes most ulcers. Interestingly, this bacterium grows better when there is less acid in the stomach. This would suggest that all the antihistamine drugs (which block stomach acid production) and antacids that people take may actually increase their risk of developing ulcers. The antihistamine drugs are among the most frequently prescribed medications.

How to take

DGL is available as chewable tablets that taste strongly of licorice. Even if you do not like the flavor of licorice, the benefits to your digestive system will probably keep you taking this supplement. Most of the DGL supplements on the market contain a small amount of fructose (extracted fruit sugar) to make the licorice flavor palatable, but it is also available without sweetener.

For best results, chew one or two tablets of DGL before each meal, or take one or two any time that you feel symptoms of acid indigestion.

Grapefruit Seed Extract

There are substances in grapefruit and other citrus seeds that have strong antifungal properties. That is, they kill yeast (fungus), often better than the medications used for the same purpose (for example, Nystatin®). Since many people have an overgrowth of the yeasts that are normally present in the intestinal tract, grapefruit seed extract is often helpful with a variety of symptoms. These symptoms are related to what is known as chronic candidiasis, which is *not* an infection, but an *overgrowth*.

Remember, these yeasts (or *Candida albicans*) are normally in your intestines, although as yet we do not know if they perform any useful functions. They do compete with the known friendly bacteria, such as *Lactobacillus acidophilus* and *Bifidobacterium bifidum*.

The overabundant intestinal yeasts release many toxins (called *mycotoxins*), which may give you a variety of systemic symptoms, including headaches, fatigue, depression, poor immune function, recurrent vaginal yeast infections and digestive disturbances. These symptoms occur even though the yeasts do *not* leave the intestines to colonize other tissues. This distinction has confused many patients and has led many physicians to dismiss intestinal yeasts as a cause of systemic symptoms. (Serious systemic yeast *infections* do occur in debilitated patients with severe immune dysfunction, cancer or other systemic diseases—but this is a different situation.)

How to take

Grapefruit seed extract is available as a liquid or in capsules containing powder. The liquid is awkward and has a strong taste, and it must be diluted to prevent local irritation of the mucous membranes. A few drops in a glass of water is still quite a strong preparation.

I recommend the capsules for convenience and to avoid any local mucous membrane irritation. They are available in 100-mg capsules, and usually one or two capsules twice daily is sufficient. Sometimes an additional dose is helpful.

Lactobacilli

Although not a botanical or flavonoid, it is appropriate to discuss the friendly intestinal flora with the grapefruit seed extract, since both help the treatment of intestinal yeast overgrowth. These are the bacteria that are present in yogurts if they *contain* live cultures, which should be clearly stated on the label. If the label says, "*made* with live cultures," it does not say whether they were killlled by pasteurization *after* the yogurt was made.

The most common cause for reduction of intestinal flora is antibiotic treatments. Antibiotics are often given for repeated infections or even for the treatment of acne. If antibiotic treatment is necessary, it is wise to take some replacement flora after the treatment is finished. The usual supplements of intestinal flora contain *Lactobacillus acidophilus* and *Bifidobacterium bifidum*.

The normal flora maintain healthy intestinal function, and they also produce some vitamins, including vitamin K and some B vitamins. They are useful for the treatment of constipation or diarrhea and help manage both irritable colon and ulcerative colitis. In addition, they have antifungal, antibacterial and antiviral properties. These bacteria also produce some anticancer substances, and they help degrade some carcinogens.

The vaginal flora of healthy women are predominantly lactobacilli. Supplements of lactobacilli can prevent and treat vaginal, urinary tract and intestinal infections. These supplements may also be given intravaginally. Recurrent vaginal yeast infections are often helped by treating the overgrowth of yeast in the intestinal tract.

How to take

Intestinal flora supplements come in both powder and capsule forms. The potent forms should contain up to *ten billion organisms* per gram. Typical doses are ¼–½ teaspoon of the powder twice per day. For capsules, the usual dose is one or two capsules twice daily. Occasionally, some people report increased diarrhea from too much friendly flora supplementation.

Stinging Nettle (Urtica dioica)

The stinging nettle plant, also called common nettle, has little surface hairs that release a stinging acid when touched.

This property is lost in cooking or in processing to make supplements. The plant extract is used therapeutically as a diuretic and for its properties in relieving allergies and hay fever symptoms and its anti-inflammatory effects. It has a number of active components.

Recent studies have incorporated nettle into regimens for treatment of prostate enlargement, not because it shrinks the prostate, but because it relieves the urethral and bladder irritation that increase urgency and frequency.

How to take

The amount of nettle used for prostate enlargement ranges from 250 to 750 mg per day. Similar doses have helped patients with allergies, usually in divided doses, taken as needed for hay fever when the symptoms occur.

Feverfew

Feverfew has a long history of use for the treatment of fevers, headaches and joint inflammation. Active principles in feverfew are called *sesquiterpenes*, such as *parthenolide*. These inhibit prostaglandin production, leading to a reduction of inflammation. It is this anti-inflammatory property that may help treat arthritis. Feverfew also lowers histamine release.

Recent studies have documented the value of feverfew in the control of migraine headaches. As little as 25 mg twice per day has reduced both the intensity and the frequency of migraine headaches. It probably produces some of its effects as a result of alterations in serotonin production. Excess serotonin production by blood platelets can trigger constriction of the arteries. Migraines are possibly related to this constriction and subsequent relaxation of these blood vessels, but the mechanisms are not yet clear.

How to take

Feverfew capsules are available in a variety of sizes. You can use the 380-mg capsules of freeze-dried leaves, but the level of the active components is quite variable, and the therapeutic value will vary with it. I usually recommend the standardized herbal extract, with a consistent 0.1–0.5% parthenolides. I suggest a 250-mg capsule twice per day.

Gugulipids

Gugulipids are derived from gugulow, an extract from the gugul tree, which grows only in particular areas of India. It has a long folk history in Ayurvedic medicine, and recent scientific evidence shows that it can lower total serum cholesterol levels while increasing the level of good HDL cholesterol. It has also helped with weight loss.

It is not clear how it works, but some people have responded remarkably well to supplements of this botanical, even if they are not strictly following healthy dietary practices. It may work by stimulation of thyroid function, but the exact mechanisms are not yet clear.

How to take

There are capsules of gugulow containing 340 mg of plant extract with 0.4% essential oils. There are also capsules of 250 mg gugulipid standardized extracts, containing 2.5% of the *gugusterones*. The usual dose is one or two capsules twice or three times per day.

Hawthorne Berry

As with many other herbs, hawthorne berries contain a number of anthocyanidins and other flavonoids. Research shows that they can lower blood pressure by dilating blood vessels, improve the cardiovascular function of patients with congestive heart failure, and reduce angina.

Hawthorne also has many of the other properties of anthocyanidin flavonoids, such as reducing allergy reactions and improving the strength of capillaries. Because of the dilation of blood vessels, it may help with Raynaud's phenomenon (spasms of the blood vessels in the hands).

How to take

Capsules containing standardized extract of hawthorne berry (2% standard) usually contain 100–250 mg of extract. Typical doses for congestive heart failure would be 250 mg, twice per day. Higher doses are sometimes recommended, but when comprehensive health promotion programs are initiated, and other effective supplements are included, it is often unnecessary to use the higher level of any one supplement.

Cranberry

Cranberries contain several substances that are thought to be clinically effective in treatment of urinary tract infections (cystitis). It is not clear which specific substances are the active components or exactly how they work, but both studies and reports from many patients confirm the value of cranberry supplements in controlling cystitis and urethritis. However, it is important to have a urine culture to diagnose urinary infections, and it may be essential to take the appropriate antibiotic for treatment. It is important not to let urinary infections go untreated because of the danger of developing a kidney infection. Cranberry may work by preventing bacteria from sticking to the bladder mucosal membrane.

Unfortunately, most commercial cranberry juice contains a large amount of sugar, and you have to drink quite a bit for it to be effective. These quantities of refined sugar are themselves detrimental to your immune system, making it more difficult to fight off infections. There is some unsweetened cranberry juice available at health food stores, but it is quite tart. If it is diluted with water and mixed with a small amount of fruit juice it can be palatable without enough sugar to adversely affect the immune system.

There are capsules of cranberry powder available for supplemental use. These are what I usually recommend for urinary infections, in addition to extra vitamin C. (I also prescribe antibiotics as needed.)

How to take

Cranberry powder is commonly available as 425-mg capsules. For most urinary infections, I suggest taking two capsules two or four times per day. If you are drinking the unsweetened juice, you may need up to one pint to be effective. This can be spread throughout the day. Sometimes a maintenance dose of cranberry supplements can prevent recurrence of infections.

Chapter 10

Practical Guidelines: Buying and Taking Supplements

When I recommend supplements, I often hear questions about where to get them and what brands to buy. How do you avoid being misled by unscrupulous manufacturers or overzealous sales pitches? Antagonists to dietary supplements sometimes leave you with the false impression that all manufacturers are disreputable. Nothing could be further from the truth. In my experience, most supplement manufacturers are reliable and honest, and *they depend on good results from their products to generate repeat sales.*

Manufacturers and Retailers

Most manufacturers follow Good Manufacturing Practices (GMPs), and you should make sure they do before purchasing their products. The purpose of GMPs is to assure that what is on the label is in the product; that the product disintegrates and is bioavailable and unadulterated. Ask your retailer to find out from their manufacturers or suppliers. You can usually find retail products at health food stores, through mail-order channels and in professional offices. I have a lot of experience with supplements sold through professional offices. They are usually of high quality and are designed by the practitioners for their own method of practice. Practitioners sometimes have their own brand label, but most of the products will be similar to those of other practitioners and comparable to retail products. It is true that practitioners sometimes will charge higher prices for their products than retail store prices, assuming that they are more convenient for their clients, but they should not be markedly different from the products you can buy through other channels. Sometimes professional products are less expensive than those from other sources.

There are also good name brands available at health food stores, and some of the larger stores have their own in-house brand labels. Several mail-order sources supply brand names similar to the ones in health food stores, and some of the larger mail-order companies also have their own labels. Like the manufacturers, they also are dependent on good results to generate repeat business. What you need to know is that *virtually all of the raw materials for dietary supplements are made in bulk by a few manufacturers.* They are then purchased by supplement "manufacturers" who only tablet, encapsulate and affix their own label to the products before sending them to distributors or retail outlets.

Be Wary of Claims

What this means most of the time is that the hyperbolic claims for particular brands are exaggerated, even though the ingredients are what they claim to be and do what they are supposed to. Some companies claim that their brand of "vitamin Z" is superior because of the form, or because it is "all natural," or it is combined with "synergistic nutrients" or herbs. Most of the time the additional dietary factors that are present are there in such small quantities that they have only a token presence—not enough to be therapeutic.

Some companies will say that their product is highly researched and tested, but when you look at the research papers that they provide, the studies refer to the basic nutrient ingredient (such as folic acid or beta-carotene) not to their particular brand. In these cases, I agree that their beta-carotene is probably healthy and of great benefit, but so are many others on the market that are just as good and usually much less expensive.

Multilevel Marketing

In my experience, most of the time the exaggerated claims are made by multilevel marketing companies. These are companies that market through a pyramid of distributors, each of whom takes a percentage of the sale. The distributors are usually just customers who want to take advantage of the "wholesale" prices that are offered to those who sign up. Some of these distributors then go on to take advantage of the business opportunity of selling retail and signing up distributors under them. They then get a percentage of the new distributor's sales, and so on down the line.

The companies' home offices often leave the impression with distributors that their product is special in a way that is not justified by research. The distributors then go off into the market and, sometimes innocently, make these unjustified claims. Again, these claims are almost invariably exaggerated and used to mark up the price of the product beyond the value of the ingredients. Always be wary if a company claims that their supplement of 2 mg is equal to 30 mg from another source. There is no basis for this claim.

Multilevel marketing companies almost always admit that their retail price is high, but you can become a distributor and get the product "wholesale." Unfortunately their wholesale price is usually still higher than comparable products sold through normal retail outlets. If you mark something up enough, a good discount still leaves you with a high price. Because of the multiple levels of distributors who take a cut from all sales, it is almost essential that the end-user price be elevated compared to other sources. To be fair, the companies claim that they save on marketing and advertising. They do less national advertising because of the zeal of distributors. This may be true, but it seems that they are not passing such savings on to the consumer.

What to Look for in Pricing

My advice is to seek a reliable mail-order, health food store or professional line of products, and check that the company uses GMPs in manufacturing. You can ask the sellers, who should be able to find out from the companies if they do not already know. Also, make sure that they are hypoallergenic and that there are no extraneous ingredients such as artificial flavor, colors or preservatives in the products. Although some of these may be safe, some of them are not, and their presence is a sign that the manufacturers are not as concerned with quality.

There have been in the past, and may still be, some very cheap mail-order supplements that did not meet the potency claims made on the label. This is much less likely now, but it is still possible. If a price looks too good to be true, it probably is. For example, if you price several reliable brands at between $9 and $12 per hundred capsules, and you find the same ingredients for $4–$6 per hundred, you need to be very suspicious. On the other hand, if you find the same product for $19, you should also be aware that you may be paying too much.

Most dietary supplement suppliers are very competitive (except for multilevel marketing prices, which are high), and a below-cost item may not meet label claim or on occasion may be made with inferior raw ingredients. These may have contamination problems or problems with solubility. Synthetic vitamin E, for example, is much cheaper than the natural form, but the molecule is slightly different, and contains only the alpha-tocopherol, not the beta, gamma or delta forms found in "mixed, natural tocopherols." That information should be on the label. The most likely supplements to be a problem are the most expensive ones, such as coenzyme Q10 or proanthocyanidins, or non-standardized herbs being sold for low prices compared to the standardized products.

Timed Release?

Most "timed-release" products are not worth the extra money that you may spend on them. In fact, they may even be less effective than the plain variety. For example, in order to achieve the best effects with vitamin C, especially in viral infections, you sometimes need a very high blood level. These levels are more difficult to achieve with timed-release pills, because of their slow dissolution and absorption.

Occasionally timed-release pills are not properly timed, so that the tablet does not disintegrate and dissolve in time or in the right place to be well absorbed from the intestinal tract. Most plain supplements are fairly well absorbed and utilized, so a slow-release form is unnecessary. There are two exceptions to this that are worth mentioning. One is vitamin B3, or niacin, which can cause a temporary flush of the skin, but is less likely to do so in timed-release form.

(Remember, however, that the timed-release form is more likely to cause liver problems in some people.) The other valuable timed-release supplement is iron, which often causes some constipation and indigestion in plain form. It is usually better tolerated as timed-release iron fumarate. The common drug-store variety, iron sulfate, seems to be the worst for causing constipation.

Combination Supplements

Except for a multivitamin and a few simple combinations, it is better to take your individual nutrients in separate pills. This makes it easier to change the dose of one nutrient without having to alter many others at the same time. It is almost invariably less expensive to take separate nutrients, but you can expect to take from six to 10 pills twice per day for a comprehensive, basic supplement program. This is assuming you are healthy. If you have a health problem, you might end up taking 10–15 pills twice a day. For vigorous longevity programs, you may end up taking quite a few more.

Manufacturers make specific combinations to distinguish their product from others—to establish a position, or "market niche." Such "exclusive" products can often command a higher price. Do not be drawn in by their exaggerated claims. A product may well have all of the claimed benefits, but is it worth the price? Compare the ingredients (mg to mg, or IU to IU) and the price. Once you have an established program with which you are satisfied, then you might find a few combinations that meet your needs, and you can use them to reduce the number of pills that you take.

If you find that a particular brand works for you and it is reasonably priced, stay with it. You might want to ask your health practitioner for advice. If you haven't tried comparable products, you would be wise to shop around for price. Ask how long a brand has been on the market. Most of the reliable companies have been around for a while. (Of course, new reliable companies do appear in the marketplace.)

There was a time when there were more unscrupulous companies selling dietary supplements, but as the industry has matured they have formed trade groups to help monitor each other. Also, the consumer is becoming more sophisticated at evaluating supplements, because there are frequent articles in the newspapers and magazines on the topic. Companies now have to keep on their toes if they are to stay in business, and they have to sell effective, competitive products.

When to Take Supplements

Most of the time, it is a good idea to take supplements with food. Nutrients occur in nature as combinations with each other and with other substances in foods. Generally, they work together in digestion, absorption and other physiological processes. Also, it is much easier on the digestion to take supplements with food. Supplements are concentrated, and sometimes they can cause digestive upset or abdominal discomfort when taken in large doses on an empty stomach.

Single nutrients, such as vitamin C can usually be taken at any time, in almost any dose, without upsetting your system. Taking a drink of pure vitamin C powder mixed with dilute fruit juice is actually refreshing, and it is an easy way to take a large dose.

Sometimes, there is antagonism or competition for absorption between different nutrients, such as copper and zinc, or in utilization, for example, iron and vitamin E. However, these are usually not sufficient to be a serious concern when taking large doses of supplements.

There are some exceptions to this rule. For example, some of the amino acids are better utilized for specific purposes when taken separately from foods. (See Chapter 8.) My recommendation is not to worry too much about such combinations; they are minor, and worrying about them makes supplement programs confusing and inconvenient. If you do not remember to take things, they are not going to do you any good.

You may have concerns about swallowing so many pills if you are on many different supplements. If you have difficulty, it is easiest to take them with a thicker liquid, such as tomato juice or a blended fruit and yogurt smoothee. This usually makes it easy to open the throat for swallowing and coats the pills, making it easier for them to go down. After you are able to take them this way, it becomes easy to swallow many pills at one time, even with plain water, but be careful. (One of my patients uses this trick—just before taking the liquid for the pills she says to herself, "I am really thirsty." She says it helps the pills go down.)

What About Pregnancy?

Most pregnant women need extra nutrition, and most physicians will recommend at least some dietary supplements. As stated before, folic acid is essential for the prevention of some birth defects, and other nutrients are helpful in preventing toxemia of pregnancy (see B6 and magnesium). Some supplements are helpful in reducing morning sickness of pregnancy, especially pyridoxine (vitamin B6).

Most of the nutrients on basic supplement programs are helpful during pregnancy and are often recommended by obstetricians. Extra iron and calcium are useful additions to a routine supplement program. The only caution is taking too much vitamin A during the first 3 months. Anything above 10,000 IU may be too much, but this only applies to preformed vitamin A, not to beta-carotene.

How to Store Supplements

You do not need to take special precautions when storing most dietary supplements. It is usually sufficient to keep them on a shelf in a pantry or on the kitchen counter. Most of the products are quite stable if kept in dry, room-temperature conditions. As with any food, do not leave them for prolonged periods in a hot car or in a closed carrier out in the sun, where they will easily get overheated.

Sometimes people are tempted to put their supplements in the refrigerator, but this is not a good idea. Every time you open a bottle of cold supplement pills in a warm external environment, there will be some condensation on the surface of the pills that remain in the bottle. Eventually, they will become wet and sticky, or they will actually begin to dissolve, depending on how much they attract moisture. An exception is some supplements of intestinal flora (lactobacilli or bifidobacteria), which sometimes keep better in the cold.

For the same reason, do not keep your supplements in the bathroom (not that you were really tempted to do so). It gets too humid with all the showering to keep them dry and fresh. The best place for storage is probably the kitchen, since it is usually dry, and it is convenient, since you will mostly take your supplements with meals.

How Long Do They Keep?

It is not a good idea to keep supplements for a long time after they have been opened. Although some are quite stable in a dry environment, there is inevitably some oxidation and loss of potency. The amount of loss depends on the particular nutrient. Many of the supplements are quite stable, and last for years if kept cool and dry. Minerals do not deteriorate with time.

With some products, the surface of the pill will change color when some components oxidize. When this happens, the surface of the tablets usually becomes darker and mottled. You should discard these tablets. You can also see this kind of discoloration inside of some two-part capsules, and you should discard these also. (Some products normally have a mixed-color surface, and you should get to know what they look like when you first buy them so you will know when they change.)

The best course of action is to buy what you need for a 1- to 3-month period or up to 6 or 8 months if it is more convenient, and store unopened bottles in a cool (but not necessarily refrigerated), dark room. If you buy a large amount, you may keep the unopened bottles in the refrigerator, but be sure to bring them to room temperature before opening them, and don't store them in the fridge once they have been opened.

Multi-compartment Storage Boxes

One last note that will make it easier for you to take supplements if you are taking more than a few: There are multi-compartment storage containers, similar to fishing tackle or sewing boxes, but with a rubber gasket seal to keep out air. They come with six to 16 chambers, to hold a number of different supplements. Label each chamber unless you clearly recognize the different supplements. If you have too many for the box, you can mix two in one chamber as long as you recognize the difference.

The advantage of having one of these multi-compartment boxes is that you only have to open one lid each time you want to take your supplements. Since you might be taking many different products at one time, this is an enormous time saver. And if you have arthritis, it will help reduce the stress on your hands from opening so many bottles so frequently.

Another way to accomplish this is to purchase some empty pharmacy vials and set aside some time to fill up a 1-week supply of morning and evening doses all at once. It is a good idea to have different size vials for your morning and evening for recognition, in case the doses are different.

Both of these methods have one further advantage, in that the original storage bottle for each supplement is opened less frequently, reducing exposure of the main supply to air and humidity. You should not have great difficulty keeping supplements safely.

Chapter 11

Your Personal Supplement Program

With all this information, how do you go about setting up a personal dietary supplement program for yourself? There are so many different supplements and so many approaches to health programs that it may seem confusing. Many sources of information on supplements will tell you of the value of some of them, but will leave you unsure of where to begin your own program. Because of this confusion, many people give up in frustration, but *it is important to your health to get started now.*

In this chapter you will find some basic guidelines and some sample programs for health enhancement and preventive medicine. You will also find some sample treatment programs for specific conditions. Consider them as guidelines, not prescriptions. When reading these recommendations, always keep in mind that your particular needs may require more or less than what you see here. This is for both the specific supplements you might need and the amounts of any one of them.

If you are a physician, remember: *it is an error to try to treat diagnoses rather than people.* Everyone is an individual, and frequently health problems occur in combinations. There are also specific life situations that demand personal attention in designing a health program. Keep this in mind when recommending supplements or any other health program for your patients. More physician training is available in this field, especially through the *American College for Advancement in Medicine.*

Supplements Are Supplements

First, a reminder that supplements are just that: additions to a healthy diet and support for many health practices. They neither replace good foods nor eliminate the need for exercise and stress management, laughter and a positive attitude. I have often known people who think that supplements could relieve them of the discipline required to change their health habits. No one health practice cures or prevents all illness and degeneration, even though any one of them will help to some degree.

Second, remember to *keep any health program simple enough to follow.* If you make it too complex, chances are you will fall off the program and lose all of the potential benefits. Take any dietary supplements at breakfast, dinner or bedtime, unless you have unusual discipline and can remember lunchtime doses. There is some small benefit in absorption of nutrients from dividing your intake of water-soluble supplements into three daily doses, but *not* if you do not remember to take them.

If you do not eat breakfast, it is time to reconsider your health habits, since breakfast is an important meal. Even if it is just a piece of fruit with some whole grain toast and a few almonds, or some whole grain cereal, try to eat something to start your day. If you absolutely cannot face food before noon, take the first dose of supplements with your lunch, and the second dose with your evening meal at least 6–8 hours later.

General Prevention

For general preventive medicine, you may wish to start with the basic supplements essential for health promotion, assuming you are in good health. These would be the *Basic Multiple* formula, some extra vitamins C and E, and probably some natural carotenes. The extra E and carotenes can be taken any time of day, since they are fat soluble and not rapidly turned over. If you do not divide the water-soluble supplements into at least two doses per day, some of them will be less well-absorbed and excreted more rapidly. They will still benefit you, but perhaps not as much. If you are concerned that you might not tolerate some of the supplements because of unusual sensitivities, you might wish to start with one at a time for a few days. If you wish, take one formula, as indicated below, for 2 or 3 days, and if there is no problem with that one add another for 2 or 3 days, and so on. The following table represents such a basic supplement program:

	AM	PM
Basic Multiple Formula	3	3
Vitamin C 1000 mg	2	2
Vitamin E 400 IU natural, mixed	1	
Natural carotenes 25,000 IU	1	

Stronger Protection

If you wish to pursue a stronger preventive medicine program, if you exercise heavily, or if you are exposed to toxic chemicals in your environment or are under unusual emotional stress, it is advisable to take extra supplements. Vitamins E and C, an essential fatty acid supplement, and a few other antioxidants, such as the mixed bioflavonoids, are

147

likely to be helpful. I would also recommend additional magnesium and some coenzyme Q10, especially if you are over 40 years old. This supplement program is represented in the following table:

	AM	PM
Basic Multiple Formula	3	3
Vitamin C 1000 mg	3	3
Bioflavonoid mix 1000 mg	1	1
Magnesium aspartate 200 mg	1	
GLA 240 mg (borage oil)	1	
Vitamin E 400 IU natural mixed	1	1
Natural carotenes 25,000 IU	1	
Coenzyme Q10 50–100 mg	1	

Vigorous Life Enhancement

For more vigorous protection from free radicals and to slow or even reverse some of the effects of aging, you will need extra dietary supplements and higher doses of some. Include additional vitamin C and magnesium, higher amounts of coenzyme Q10, and some more phytochemical flavonoids, as reflected in the following table:

	AM	PM
Basic Multiple Formula	3	3
Vitamin C 1000 mg	4	4
Bioflavonoid mix 1000 mg	1	1
Quercetin 400 mg	1	
Magnesium aspartate 200 mg	1	1
GLA 240 mg (borage oil)	1	
Vitamin E 400 IU natural mixed	1	1
Natural carotenes 25,000 IU	1	1

	AM	PM
Coenzyme Q10 100–200 mg	1	
Proanthocyanidins 50 mg mixed	1	1

As You Age

These previous programs are by no means the most extreme programs that some people are following. As you age, for example into your fifties and sixties, you may wish to add those nutrients that further help to protect memory, vision, liver function, and gastrointestinal health, in addition to preventing cancer, diabetes, heart disease, and stroke. This further list of supplements might include extra selenium, *Ginkgo biloba*, silymarin, bilberry, glutamine, melatonin, and carnitine. Admittedly, this is a vigorous program with many pills to take and greater expense. However, even if it were 10 dollars a day, it would be less than what some people spend on cigarettes, coffee, colas, hotdogs, and doughnuts! The following table represents such a program:

	AM	PM
Basic Multiple Formula	3	3
Vitamin C 1000 mg	4	4
Bioflavonoid mix 1000 mg	1	1
Quercetin 400 mg	1	1
Magnesium aspartate 200 mg	1	1
GLA 240 mg (from borage oil)	1	
Vitamin E 400 IU natural mixed	1	1
Natural carotenes 25,000 IU	1	1
Coenzyme Q10 200 mg	1	
L-Glutamine 500 mg	2	2
L-Carnitine 250 mg	2	2
Ginkgo biloba extract 60 mg	1	1

	AM	PM
Bilberry 100 mg	1	1
Selenium 200 mcg	1	
Proanthocyanidins 50 mg mixed	1	1
Silymarin 150 mg (80% standardized)	1	1
Melatonin 3 mg		1–2

If you have specific health problems, it is important to have them diagnosed first. If they are chronic degenerative conditions, or your health practitioner says, "Well, what do you expect at your age?" then it is time to consider some of the therapeutic supplements that are described in the previous chapters. (You might also try to find a more responsive health practitioner.)

Your attempt to enhance your health is not a substitute for diagnosis and proper treatment of medical conditions. You can, however, enhance your health and increase the likelihood of success of any other treatment regimen. You will also probably decrease the side effects of medication and increase the rate of healing after surgery or other treatment.

Treatment Programs

When patients come to me for advice about specific medical problems, they usually have been told that they need medication or surgery, and they are seeking ways to avoid those treatments. Sometimes they have already tried medications, which have produced significant side effects.

Usually, they have many treatment alternatives but they have no information about their choices. One example of effective alternatives is the reduction in blood pressure that meditation produces. Others are the dietary changes and exercise programs that lead to lowered cholesterol. Since the medical treatments for these two conditions are often more dangerous than the problems, it is worth seeking safer alternatives.

Dr. Dean Ornish has shown that patients with heart disease can often avoid surgery and reverse their heart disease with a combination of a low-fat diet, meditation, and exercise. Norman Cousins healed his ankylosing spondylitis (a form of arthritis of the spine) with laughter and high doses of vitamin C. He wrote about his experience in the *New England Journal of Medicine,* and followed this article with a book, *The Anatomy of an Illness.* Many patients have cured their digestive disturbances simply by avoiding certain foods.

Over and over, we are seeing the results of lifestyle changes in health care. A recent scientific medical conference put on by the American College for Advancement in Medicine was entitled: *Lifestyle Medicine—Medicine for the Nineties.* Researchers and physicians both attended and taught at this scientific meeting. Much of it related to the role of dietary supplements in medical therapy.

Dietary supplements are among the safest and most effective choices in health care. They are almost free of side effects, they are easy to take, they are relatively inexpensive, and they usually enhance many life functions besides the specific condition for which they are being given. Here are some examples of how nutritionally oriented physicians might use supplements as part of the treatment for some specific health problems. These are suggestions that are supported in the medical literature and in the experience of many physicians.

Remember that these are examples, not prescriptions for you, and the supplement list is in addition to many other health practices. Other supplements may be helpful, and you may not need all of these to get results. For more information on any one supplement, look for its description in previous chapters. No one program is appropriate for everybody, but these suggestions are good starting points from which individual programs can be modified.

Hypertension (High Blood Pressure)

High blood pressure, even if mild, is associated with an increased risk of vascular diseases, including heart disease and stroke. The pressures are read as the *systolic*, which is the first number (when the heart pumps), and the *diastolic*, the second number (between beats). Disease risks are increased whenever the diastolic pressure is above 80. Such elevations are related to excess salt, sugar, caffeine and animal fat in the diet, and obesity, which are all very common in the United States. It is also related to stress, smoking, alcohol consumption, and sedentary lifestyles.

Hypertension usually has no symptoms in early stages. It is common for blood pressure to rise as people age, but this is not physiologically normal or healthy; it is considered normal by physicians because it is so common. The following is a preliminary program, which can be easily enhanced if it is not working adequately to lower blood pressure. Of course, if the problem is severe or nonresponsive, medication may be in order. If there are other complicating conditions, other supplements may be helpful.

	AM	PM
Basic Multiple Formula	3	3
Vitamin C 1000 mg	3	3
Pyridoxine (B6) 250 mg	1	
Magnesium aspartate 200 mg	1	1
GLA 240 mg (from borage oil)		1
Vitamin E 400 IU natural mixed	1	1

	AM	PM
Coenzyme Q10 100 mg	1	
Garlic, deodorized, 500 mg	1	1
EPA fish oil	2	2
Taurine 500 mg	2	2

Allergies and Asthma

Since allergies and asthma are so often related, and the therapeutic supplements are so similar, they are linked in the discussion. Allergic symptoms may be as simple as hay fever or sinus congestion. They may be precipitants of sinus infections. Asthmatic wheezing is more serious. Stress reduction frequently plays a large role in the management of asthma, and attacks may be precipitated by stress. Food allergies are also common complicating factors.

Asthma may be severe, and it is unwise to stop your medication unless symptoms are well controlled. Supplement doses may need to be increased, such as extra quercetin or nettle, to manage allergic responses. Occasionally, someone is sensitive to a specific supplement. This is unpredictable, so be on the lookout for reactions. The most valuable supplements include:

	AM	PM
Basic Multiple Formula	3	3
Vitamin C 1000 mg	3	3
Quercetin 400 mg	1	1
Pyridoxine (B6) 250 mg	1	
Magnesium aspartate 200 mg	1	1
GLA 240 mg (from borage oil)	1	
Vitamin E 400 IU natural mixed	1	1
Coenzyme Q10 100–200 mg	1	

153

	AM	PM
Proanthocyanidins 50 mg mixed	1	1
Nettle 250 mg	2	2

Angina/Hardening of the Arteries

Arteriosclerotic heart disease and other vascular diseases result from the buildup of plaque (fatty, fibrous and calcified tissue) in the coronary arteries and the arteries to the brain, abdomen, pelvic organs and legs. As mentioned earlier, it may be caused or reversed by many lifestyle habits. Common symptoms of heart disease include chest tightness or pain, which may radiate to the left arm, jaw, or chin; shortness of breath; and fatigue. Sometimes the symptom is described as a pressure sensation, or even as heartburn or indigestion.

Cerebral artery disease leads to faintness, loss of mental function, and strokes. Hardening of the arteries to the pelvic organs can lead to sexual dysfunction, and leg arterial disease leads to pain in the calves on walking and poor circulation to the feet, which may end up as gangrene.

It is essential to have a good cardiologic and vascular evaluation in addition to any health enhancement program. Depending on the symptoms and history, the supplement program may be quite variable, but the following list includes those supplements that are most likely to be beneficial:

	AM	PM
Basic Multiple Formula	3	3
Vitamin C 1000 mg	3	3
Magnesium aspartate 200 mg	1	1
GLA 240 mg (from borage oil)	1	

	AM	PM
Vitamin E 400 IU natural mixed	1	1
Natural carotenes 25,000 IU	1	
Coenzyme Q10 200 mg	1	
L-Carnitine 250 mg	2	2
Ginkgo biloba extract 60 mg	1	1
Niacin-inositol 400 mg	2	2
Proanthocyanidins 50 mg mixed	1	1
Taurine 500 mg	2	2

Digestive Disorders

There are many varieties of digestive problems, including inflammatory diseases (Crohn's disease, ulcerative colitis, diverticulitis), acid indigestion (heartburn), peptic ulcers, hiatal hernia, irritable colon, lactose intolerance, yeast overgrowth, food allergies and others. No one program is suitable for all of these digestive problems.

Some of the most commonly prescribed drugs are those that are supposed to help with acid indigestion and ulcers, but these medications are overused and often improperly prescribed. They are also common causes of serious gastrointestinal bleeding. There are many non-drug treatments that help with many gastrointestinal disorders. Some of the generally helpful dietary supplements are listed in the following table:

	AM	PM
Basic Multiple Formula	3	3
Vitamin C 1000 mg	3	3
Pyridoxine (B6) 250 mg	1	
Magnesium aspartate 200 mg	1	1
GLA 240 mg (as borage oil)	1	

155

	AM	PM
Vitamin E 400 IU natural, mixed	1	1
L-Glutamine 500 mg	3	3
Garlic deodorized 500 mg	2	2
Lactobacillus	2	2
Deglycirrhizinated licorice	chew as needed	

Premenstrual Syndrome (PMS)

Premenstrual symptoms range from mild to severe, and they include bloating, cramps, headaches, fluid retention, depression, low back pain, abdominal pressure, sugar cravings, anxiety, irritability, breast tenderness, acne, and mood swings. Some of these symptoms may also occur during the menstrual period, especially cramps, and they are often controlled by the same supplements.

For both premenstrual and menstrual symptoms, in addition to the dietary supplement program, you may need supplements of *natural progesterone*. This is the hormone, produced primarily by the ovaries, but also by the adrenal glands, that supports pregnancy and also helps to maintain and increase bone density. It also counteracts excessive estrogen stimulation.

Natural progesterone (as opposed to synthetic "progestins" such as Provera®) has no side effects and it regulates many different functions. It is particularly important to menopausal women for *increasing* bone density and managing some menopausal symptoms. (Synthetic progestins are different, and do little for bone density.) Progesterone is commonly deficient, is free of side effects, and can be taken as a supplement either orally or as a skin cream. It is wise to have a gynecologic examination before proceeding with progesterone treatment.

The following table of supplements includes those most

commonly helpful with both premenstrual syndrome and menstrual symptoms:

	AM	PM
Basic Multiple Formula	3	3
Vitamin C 1000 mg	2	2
Pyridoxine (B6) 250 mg	1	
Magnesium aspartate 200 mg	1	1
GLA 240 mg (from borage oil)	1	
Vitamin E 400 IU natural mixed	1	1
Flaxseed oil, 1–2 tbsp daily, or		
EPA 1000 mg	2	2

Candidiasis (Yeast Overgrowth)

The overgrowth of yeast in the intestinal tract was mentioned in the section on grapefruit seed extract. It can lead to a variety of symptoms as a result of the toxins that yeasts produce (mycotoxins). These symptoms are the result of allergy or toxins, not yeast in the blood stream or organs. It is sometimes difficult to reduce the intestinal yeast population but there are several dietary supplements that can help.

In addition to the supplements, it is important to reduce dietary and medical sources of yeast growth stimulants, such as antibiotics, hormones, and a high intake of sugar. Hormones or antibiotics may be necessary for medical reasons, but the resulting yeast overgrowth needs to be controlled. Of course, refined, white sugar is always avoidable, with a little determination, if you really want to keep it out of your diet.

Although they may be combined with medications when indicated, the following supplements are commonly used to help control the yeast overgrowth:

	AM	PM
Grapefruit seed extract	2	2
Lactobacillus acidophilus capsules	2	2
Garlic (deodorized) 500 mg	2	2
GLA 240 mg (as borage oil)	1	1

I often recommend a mixture of *Lactobacillus acidophilus* with the *Bifidobacterium bifidum*, either in capsule or powder form. This combination helps both the large and small intestines. The dose of powder is usually ½ tsp twice per day at the start of treatment and ¼ tsp twice per day after some improvement. In addition to these specifics, I would recommend that you take the usual general health supplements and immune enhancers such as the following:

	AM	PM
Basic Multiple Formula	3	3
Vitamin C 1000 mg	3	3
Pyridoxine (B6) 250 mg	1	
Magnesium aspartate 200 mg	1	1
Vitamin E 400 IU	1	
Echinacea 250 mg	2	2

These supplements and several others may be indicated for the management of various symptoms that people with candidiasis often experience. It is important to have a proper diagnosis, in case your symptoms are from other causes.

Congestive Heart Failure

The inability of the heart muscle to pump out all of the blood that is returned through the veins is called congestive heart failure. Fluid is forced out of the blood vessels into the surrounding tissues by the back pressure. The symptoms are shortness of breath, fatigue, and other signs of heart problems.

Swelling of the legs occurs when the smaller right chamber (ventricle) of the heart is involved, but both the right and left ventricles may be involved at the same time. It is important to avoid salt in the diet to reduce excess fluid accumulation. There are several dietary supplements that can help heart failure, but it is important to have a proper diagnosis and medical management, since this can be a serious situation. Helpful supplements include:

	AM	PM
Basic Multiple Formula	3	3
Vitamin C 1000 mg	3	3
Magnesium aspartate 200 mg	1	1
Vitamin E 400 IU natural mixed	1	1
Coenzyme Q10 200 mg	1	
Taurine 500 mg	3	3
Hawthorne berry 250 mg	2	1

Again, other supplements are helpful with conditions that either cause or accompany heart failure, and they should be considered based on individual needs.

Diabetes

Diabetes mellitus (sometimes called "sugar diabetes") is a failure to properly metabolize sugar, specifically blood glucose. It results from either the reduced function of the pancreas, which produces insulin, or more commonly from inability of the cells to respond to insulin, called *insulin resistance*. Insulin is essential to move sugar out of the bloodstream into the muscles, where it can be burned for energy.

159

There are many causes of diabetes, the most common form of which is adult onset, which is almost always the result of poor health habits and being overweight. The symptoms of diabetes are excessive thirst and hunger and frequent urination. Most of the time, adult-onset diabetes does not require insulin or the oral medications that are used to control blood sugar, and most people can be taken off medication if they follow the right diet (high fiber, high complex carbohydrate, low fat) and if they exercise.

In addition to lifestyle changes, there are specific supplements that help diabetics to control their blood sugar and to prevent complications, such as eye and vascular disorders. Even Type I diabetics (juvenile type, or insulin dependent) can reduce their insulin doses with a complete approach to blood sugar management. Nonetheless, medical supervision of diabetes is usually essential, and I do not recommend trying to manage diabetes yourself. The following nutrients may contribute to sugar control and prevention or management of diabetic complications:

	AM	PM
Basic Multiple Formula	3	3
Vitamin C 1000 mg	3	3
Bioflavonoid mix 1000 mg	1	1
Quercetin 400 mg	1	1
Magnesium aspartate 200 mg	1	1
GLA 240 mg (from borage oil)	1	
Vitamin E 400 IU natural mixed	1	1
Coenzyme Q10 200 mg	1	
Ginkgo biloba extract 60 mg	1	1
Bilberry 100 mg	1	1
Chromium 200 mcg	2	2
Proanthocyanidins 50 mg mixed	1	1
Silymarin 150 mg (80% standardized)	1	1

Fatigue

One of the most common complaints in any medical practice is fatigue (usually for both the patient and the doctor). There are many causes of persistent fatigue, as opposed to simply being tired from exercise or a heavy work load. There may be a serious medical disorder such as anemia, diabetes, heart disease, chronic fatigue/immune-dysfunction syndrome (also called CFIDS), and infection.

Some chronic everyday problems may also cause significant ongoing fatigue, such as stress, dietary imbalance, food allergy, nutritional deficiency, environmental toxicity, low blood sugar (hypoglycemia), and low-grade depression. Sometimes the problem is as simple as a lack of adequate exercise or boredom. There are some general principles for reducing fatigue after eliminating any of the serious medical conditions as the underlying cause.

Again, eating properly, exercising, and reducing emotional stressors can help increase your energy. Avoiding food allergens and environmental toxins helps reduce exposure to the chemical stressors. A general dietary supplement is often adequate to help fatigue due to nutritional imbalances or borderline deficiencies.

Do not ignore the need to find out if persistent fatigue is the result of a serious medical problem. Treatment may require medical management in addition to lifestyle change and dietary supplements. The following supplement program often helps with fatigue from many causes:

	AM	PM
Basic Multiple Formula	3	3
Vitamin C 1000 mg	2	2
Niacin, timed release, 250 mg	1	1
Magnesium aspartate 200 mg	1	1

	AM	PM
GLA 240 mg (from borage oil)	1	
Vitamin E 400 IU natural, mixed	1	1
Coenzyme Q10 100 mg	1	
Chromium 200 mcg	1	1
L-Glutamine 500 mg	1	1
L-Carnitine 250 mg	2	2

Headaches

As with fatigue, there are many causes of headaches. The most common problems are tension or stress-related headaches and migraine headaches. Assuming there are no brain tumors, hypertension, or infections, such as meningitis, which can cause acute headaches, treatment with lifestyle changes and dietary supplements is often effective.

Migraines are called vascular headaches because they result from blood vessel spasms. There are many triggers that can precipitate migraine headaches. Common ones are caffeine, alcohol (especially red wine), chocolate, and sugar. Food allergies can also lead to a migraine, as can exposure to bright or flickering lights, lack of sleep or emotional and psychological stress.

Most effective programs for headache control, other than drug treatments, rely on prevention. The pain-killer medications that are often used to treat migraines (Advil®, Motrin®, ibuprofen—all of which have the same active ingredient) have actually been shown to increase the severity and frequency of the headaches, possibly through some rebound effect, leading to more use of the medications. The following supplement program is often effective for the drug-free management of migraines and may also help the treatment of other headaches:

	AM	PM
Basic Multiple Formula	3	3
Vitamin C 1000 mg	2	2
Pyridoxine 250 mg	1	
Magnesium aspartate 200 mg	1	1
Niacin, timed release, 250 mg	1	1
GLA 240 mg (from borage oil)	1	
Vitamin E 400 IU natural mixed	1	
Ginkgo biloba extract 60 mg	1	1
Feverfew 250 mg standardized	1	1

Arthritis

Inflammation or deterioration of the joints, with progressive destruction of the joint cartilage, is responsible for much of the disability of the elderly, although it also affects younger people. As the cartilage gets worn away, the bones of the joints rub on each other and cause varying degrees of pain.

Rheumatoid arthritis is the result of connective tissue destruction by immune complexes formed when the immune system attacks the body's own tissue. This is called *autoimmunity,* which is poor regulation (or *dysregulation*) of immune function, not simply increased activity. Some dietary supplements that enhance immune activity actually relieve rheumatoid arthritis and reduce joint destruction, since they help restore normal immune regulation.

Rheumatoid arthritis is more common in women than men, and occurs in relatively young people, most commonly starting in the thirties and forties. It is commonly associated with other immune system disorders, such as dry eye syndrome (Sjögren's syndrome) and Raynaud's phenomenon (blood vessel spasms in the hands or feet precipitated by exposure to cold).

163

Food allergies commonly play a role in causing rheumatoid arthritis. Although many physicians and the well-known national arthritis organizations often say that diet has nothing to do with arthritis, clinical experience and a number of research articles have shown otherwise. Healthy diets and avoiding food allergens are important components of arthritis treatment. Allergy tests can help pinpoint which foods to avoid. In my experience, dairy products and meats make symptoms worse, possibly because of allergy and possibly because land-animal fats can increase inflammation.

Other immune arthritis conditions include ankylosing spondylitis (arthritis of the spine) and arthritis associated with psoriasis.

Osteoarthritis, or degenerative joint disease, is more common than rheumatoid arthritis and is the result of wear and tear, infection or joint injury. After the age of 70, there is X-ray evidence of osteoarthritis in 85% of Americans, although some of them may have no symptoms. It is often helped by the same dietary supplements that relieve rheumatoid arthritis. The following supplements are often helpful for relieving symptoms and restoring joint integrity:

	AM	PM
Basic Multiple Formula	3	3
Vitamin C 1000 mg	3	3
Magnesium aspartate 200 mg	1	1
Niacinamide 500 mg	2	2
GLA 240 mg (from borage oil)	1	
EPA fish oil 1000 mg	2	2
Vitamin E 400 IU natural mixed	1	1
Glucosamine sulfate 500 mg	2	2
Proanthocyanidins 50 mg mixed	1	1

There are many reports of other supplements that sometimes help arthritis. They include extracts of sea cucumber, green-lipped mussel, and cartilage—from either shark or calf (bovine) sources. Some of my patients have reported benefits from these supplements. However, so far I am not as impressed with these products as with those in the program outlined above.

Sexual Dysfunction

The interest and ability to partake in satisfying sexual relations is an important part of living, even well into advanced years. It is an important part of loving relationships. However, there are many causes of sexual dysfunction (loss of interest or ability to take part in sex). This is sometimes called impotence in men.

Any serious medical condition, sexually transmitted diseases, depression or other psychological disorders, fatigue, overwork or simply lack of adequate sleep can lead to loss of libido (interest in sex) or ability. Hardening of the arteries to the pelvic organs may be a direct cause of sexual dysfunction. Of course, loss of interest or ability may also result from relationship problems.

Many poor health habits lead to deterioration of numerous bodily functions, and sexuality is particularly vulnerable. Smoking, obesity, high stress, lack of exercise, fatty acid imbalance (which affects hormones), and alcohol consumption are examples. Chronic problems such as candidiasis, hypoglycemia, allergies, and chronic fatigue syndrome can all lead to sexual dysfunction.

Almost any health-enhancing program of diet and exercise with basic dietary supplements can help the situation. It is also important to deal first with known medical and psychological problems. Even some of these may be helped with nutrition and dietary supplements. Remember to start by changing those harmful life habits. They will not only begin to improve your love life, but they will help to prevent the chronic and lethal degenerative diseases. An initial dietary supplement program that is likely to help is the following:

	AM	PM
Basic Multiple Formula	3	3
Vitamin C 1000 mg	2	2
Magnesium aspartate 200 mg	1	1
GLA 240 mg (as borage oil)	1	
Vitamin E 400 IU natural mixed	1	1
Coenzyme Q10 100 mg		1
Ginkgo biloba extract 60 mg	1	1

If the cause of sexual dysfunction is diabetes, heart disease, or hormonal imbalances, this program is likely to provide some help, but it is only the beginning. There are more vigorous programs for these conditions which may also help restore your sexuality and help you regain your love life.

For women with specific hormonal needs, natural progesterone supplements or natural estrogens may be valuable. For men, testosterone replacement is often part of a total program. (Even for women, there are therapeutic uses of testosterone in the treatment of heart disease and sexual dysfunction.) Hormonal supplementation with DHEA (dehydroepiandrosterone) is often of benefit to both men and women. These hormones are prescription medications, and there is a growing number of medical doctors with interest in these modern treatments.

Prostate Enlargement

Prostate enlargement (benign prostatic hypertrophy or BPH) is a common affliction in men as they age. The prostate gland sits beneath the bladder and surrounds the ure-thra, the outflow channel for urine. Symptoms of enlarge-ment include difficulty starting or stopping urination, fre-quent urination, urination at night, slow urine flow and a frequent sense of urgency to urinate. Surgery to remove some of the prostate tissue is commonly performed if the symptoms become severe enough.

There are many healthy approaches to managing pros-tate enlargement. If the symptoms are not severe, there is no risk from trying the alternatives to surgery. The new medi-cation for BPH, finasteride or Proscar®, is not as effective as the herbs and other dietary supplements, and it has poten-tial side effects. Adding pumpkin seeds to your diet is claimed to be helpful by many patients. They contain zinc and essential fatty acids that may help the condition. The following program of supplements is what I recommend for management of prostate problems:

	AM	PM
Basic Multiple Formula	3	3
Vitamin C 1000 mg	3	3
Magnesium aspartate 200 mg	1	1
GLA 240 mg (from borage oil)	1	
Vitamin E 400 IU natural mixed	1	1
Saw palmetto standardized 160 mg	1	1
Pygeum africanum 25 mg	1	1
Nettle (*Urtica dioica*) standardized 125 mg	1	1
Zinc 50 mg		1

Notes on Your Health Program

As you can see, these examples of treatment programs have many similarities. This is because many of the same supplements help a variety of health problems. Also, sometimes different supplements help the same problem, and what works will vary from one person to another. For example, individual needs for the same nutrient may vary up to 40 times.

Your response to herbs and flavonoids may be quite different from the response of your neighbor, or even that of another family member. This is the nature of biochemical individuality. Fortunately, there are also a lot of similarities among people, and this allows physicians to learn what to do for one person from our experience with another. However, the differences between people may require adjusting what we learn and adapting it for the individual. This is part of the art of healing.

These programs are useful starting points for your own needs, or if you are a physician, they can be used as foundations for developing treatment programs for your patients. You do not have to try everything at once. Whether you are just beginning a dietary supplement health program, or if you are a physician just starting in the field, you will benefit by trying only one or a few supplements and adding new ones as you become more familiar with the substances.

You know your body's individual responses better than anyone else, in some ways even better than your health practitioner, and you have to use that information to create your own health or to help your health practitioner guide you. If your practitioners are unfamiliar with this information about dietary supplements, you can help them begin to understand it by giving them this book. This will help you to become a partner in your health care.

Chapter 12

My Personal Prevention Program

I have been taking dietary supplements for 25 years. Before I started in 1970, I had the same attitude that most doctors had (and many still do today) that if you eat a balanced diet you don't need supplements. As you have seen, this is simply not true (and many doctors, and even dietitians, still do not know what a good diet is). Fortunately, I learned about supplements early in my career (and even more fortunately for me, early in my life).

I now feel as healthy as or healthier than I did when I started taking supplements at 25 years old. I have virtually no colds, normal weight, good cholesterol levels, no signs of degenerative disease, lots of energy and a sense of vitality, all of which is unusual in my age group. Part of this is surely due to my healthy, whole foods, mostly vegetarian diet (I eat no meat or chicken), part to my love of exercise, and some to my genes, but these are certainly enhanced by the supplements that I have taken over the years.

Fanatic or Realistic?

Although it seems to some people almost fanatical that I am so careful about my diet and take so many supplements, it is strange to me that *they* do not think it fanatical to drink sodas, eat potato chips and doughnuts, and gorge on ice cream, steaks and burgers. And, although my health practices seem fanatical to some, they are clearly beneficial for comprehensive health, medical treatment, and preventive medicine.

A Leaky Valve

When I was a freshman at college, a routine evaluation of all heart murmurs among first-year students, revealed that I did not have a benign murmur as had been told to me and my family all my life. Instead, I learned that I had a truly leaky aortic valve, and the doctors said that I should give up all vigorous exercise (anything more active than golf or chess!). I was told that the condition (aortic insufficiency) would most likely deteriorate with time over the next 15 to 30 years. The doctors also said that I would most likely develop congestive heart failure as the heart became unable to keep up with the greater pumping needs (always having to send a little extra out to make up for the amount that leaked back into the heart).

At the time of my diagnosis in 1962, I had no reason to doubt the validity of what the doctors were saying. Somehow, though, even accepting the diagnosis (which I have never doubted), I was unable to allow their fears for my health future to follow me into my own life. I continued, with what some doctors considered reckless abandon, to play sports (although I used their excuse notes to escape gym requirements).

Much later in life, I learned that the doctors had wanted to replace my aortic valve with a plastic one, but my parents refused to accept surgery since I was asymptomatic, and they had a healthy skepticism of excess medical treatment.

(The technology of valve replacement has improved enormously since that time, so if I ever do need a new valve, the chances of success are much greater now than they were in 1962, and I expect them to continue to improve.)

A Change of Direction

I became interested in vitamin supplements and diet through the influence of a fascinating older Norwegian psychologist/musician/nutritionist named Kaare Bolgen, who convinced me that I hadn't learned everything in medical school. At the time, this was a shocking revelation. I also developed a healthy skepticism of many medical treatments. I was a hospital resident, training in pathology, and I saw first hand in the morgue the results of many dangerous lifestyle choices, as well as the overuse of some surgical heart treatments. I had a personal interest in doing the best I could for my heart, and I developed an interest in longevity in spite of my doctors' dire predictions. This interest in true "health care," as opposed to "disease care," was soon translated into my medical practice.

My Own Health Habits

Since my exposure to the importance of dietary supplements, I have been taking them myself and recommending them for my patients (and anyone else who wants to listen). I have also run marathons, played racquetball, done long-distance bicycling trips (and more recently, taken up in-line skating). I eat a whole foods diet (especially avoiding sugar and margarines), which is mostly vegetarian (no meat or chicken), and I try to keep my stress levels in control.

In the early 1980s, I went to see another cardiologist, Dr. George Sheehan, who was a distance runner himself and a well-known writer on running. His conclusion, after evaluating my heart, was that my earlier doctors were right in their description of what "might" happen, but they had no scientific reason to claim that exercise would bring on heart failure. It might even be the case that exercise would make the situation better. Also, those cardiologists did not account for the nutrition and dietary supplements that could help strengthen and protect the heart. (Of course, that was in 1962, and there were only a few people who were aware of the relationship between diet, supplements, and disease—I was not one of them.)

Through medical school I had the same health habits as my fellow students—burgers, fries, a cola, and frequent coffee. I also only exercised periodically and knew nothing of stress control. These are the typical unhealthy habits of young people, but they are now known to lead to serious problems after the resilience of youth is dissipated and sometimes even earlier. I survived this without observable serious problems, but I continued to have several colds and flus each year.

I now take many supplements, and, as I become older, I am increasing the levels of those that protect me from the ravages of aging and free-radical damage. I am not suggesting that my own program is right for anyone else, but I am presenting it as an example of a vigorous health enhancement program that I suspect will keep me healthy well into advanced years.

No one has a way of knowing what will happen in the future, but one of the advantages of a longevity program such as mine is that it also keeps me feeling vigorous and alive in the present. Results in the present are what keep most people on track, and I am no different. As you feel better on your own program, it will reinforce your desire to stay with it.

What I Take

I take my supplements twice every day, and almost never miss a dose. If I miss the morning dose for any reason, I will take them later with my lunch. Although I vary my intake somewhat from day to day, my personal health program consists of the following basic supplements:

	AM	PM
Basic Multiple Formula	3	3
Vitamin C 1000 mg	7	6
Bioflavonoid mix 1000 mg	1	1
Quercetin 400 mg	1	1
Pyridoxine (B6) 250 mg	1	
Folic acid 20 mg	1	
Magnesium aspartate 200 mg	1	1
GLA 240 mg (borage oil)	1	
Vitamin E 400 IU natural mixed	1	1
Natural carotenes 25,000 IU	1	1
Coenzyme Q10 200 mg chewable	1	
L-Glutamine 500 mg	2	2
L-Carnitine 250 mg	2	2
Ginkgo biloba extract 60 mg	1	1
Eye nutrients/bilberry 100 mg	1	1
Special antioxidant formula	1	1
Niacin-inositol 400 mg	1	1
Selenium 200 mcg	1	
Proanthocyanidins 50 mg mixed	1	1
Saw palmetto extract 160 mg	1	1
Melatonin 3 mg		1

I take all my supplements after breakfast or supper, except that I take the melatonin at bedtime. I take the saw palmetto extract, although I have no sign of prostate enlargement, because I believe that in my age group it is good preventive medicine.

I also take some other supplements periodically, or as needed, if I feel stressed or fatigued. For example, I take two capsules of echinacea daily for 1 week periodically for enhancing immune function, or if I feel that I might be getting a virus (a rare situation these days). I also take three or four capsules of silymarin for liver cleansing on occasion. If I have been very busy and my mind is racing, I might add some GABA (gamma-aminobutyric acid), a calming neurotransmitter, to my bedtime dose of melatonin. I also take some calming herbs (passion flower, valerian, skullcap, and hops in a combination, or some kava kava) to help sleep. Sometimes I take an extra coenzyme Q10 tablet, or higher doses of L-carnitine.

As I learn about new research on dietary supplements and orthomolecular substances, I am always on the lookout for materials that might help both me and my patients to enhance our health. In addition to doing things that promote my own health, I believe in setting the example for my patients in exercise, diet, stress reduction and dietary supplementation. It is much easier to believe professionals who practice what they preach. (Since I only preach what I practice, it is easy for me to set a good example; it does not require any great virtue.) I expect to be setting the example for many years to come.

Science and Medicine

Part of what I am doing is experimental, but that does not mean that it is not documented. Science is an important method of study that always gives us new information and new ways of looking at information. The facts revealed by scientific study are never perfect. Imperfect data must always be used to draw conclusions, but we have to be open to the possibility that later information will change our view and provide new insights into the role of dietary supplements in health care—both treatment and prevention.

I do not want to wait for the final scientific word on these safe supplements. They have good research and clinical experience to back them up, and anyway, science never provides the final word—it is a dynamic search for truth that always depends on the current state of our knowledge. Right now, that knowledge says that the wisest approach to health care, along with diet, exercise and stress management, includes taking dietary supplements.

Chapter 13

Dietary Supplements: Political Pressure Cooker

In recent years, the political and bureaucratic pressures surrounding dietary supplements have exploded with new attempts by the United States Food and Drug Administration (FDA) to restrict the flow of information about them. Through a misguided fear of "snake-oil salesmen" and a mission to promote the development and safety of new drugs, the FDA has been on a vendetta against the dietary supplement industry since early in its history. They apparently see dietary supplements as a threat to patented pharmaceutical agents.

This situation in the United States has implications for other countries, since many of them take their regulatory cues from the actions of the FDA. In Norway, for example, doses of supplements beyond the RDA were at first banned, and then the government opened a chain of stores that became the only ones allowed to sell high-dose supplements. In 1994, I had an opportunity to testify at meetings in Great Britain concerning European Economic Community regulations of dietary supplement doses. The issue has not yet been resolved there. This is an ongoing struggle in many countries and seems to threaten the status quo wherever anyone wants to take charge of their own health care.

Protecting You from Information

The FDA's regulatory efforts are purportedly aimed at protecting the public from misinformation that the marketers of dietary supplements might use to sell their products. It is true that this has happened in the past and is happening, although to a lesser extent, today. However, the issue has come to the fore because in their zeal the FDA is "protecting" the public from accurate information that will do them a world of good.

The truth is, there has been an explosion of new research data showing the value of dietary supplements in almost every sphere of health care. From cancer to heart disease to AIDS to headaches, dietary supplements are being shown to be of value. They are helping people stay off drugs and they are reducing the costs of health care, in terms of both money and undesired side effects.

In spite of official opposition to supplements (from both government agencies and much of mainstream medicine), the public demand for them is growing. In response to this, the FDA has used rule making and legal maneuvering to subvert the intent of the laws that Congress passed designed to increase the flow of nutrition information to the public.

In 1992 and 1993, Congress considered bills that would restrict the ability of the FDA to skirt around the intent of the laws. During the hearings held by the Senate Labor and Human Resources Committee in 1993, the commissioner of the FDA, David Kessler, made some erroneous statements about supplements. He also put on a show of some bottles of dietary supplements that he claimed were "misbranded" because they made health claims.

Any health claims for dietary supplements were against the regulations of the FDA if they were made by supplement manufacturers or distributors, even if they were truthful and not misleading and even if they were the same health claims that other agencies of the US government were making. For example, if the US Public Health Service suggested folic acid supplements for pregnant women, it was illegal for a company marketing folic acid to quote that agency in its promotional literature.

The bill then being considered, the *Dietary Supplement and Health Education Act*, eventually passed despite the opposition of some vehement protectors of the FDA. However, many of the most important sections of the Senate version of the bill, which would allow the easiest public access to supplement information, were deleted before the bill was passed by the House of Representatives. This was the result of compromises with powerful committee chairpersons.

As of this writing, in 1995, efforts are underway to correct some of the omissions of the final version of the bill as passed into law. Other committees are considering stricter oversight of the FDA, in order to prevent them from making laws through "regulations" and interpretation.

I testified at those 1993 Senate hearings and had to depart from my prepared testimony in order to address some of the misinformation presented by the director of the FDA. I then submitted to the committee some written follow-up testimony which included most of the statements that I felt compelled to present ad lib. Although I have seen it many times, I am always surprised when scientific information is misrepresented for political purposes. Here is the original version of my testimony, and the follow-up testimony.

Senate Testimony

My name is Michael Janson. I am a physician in Massachusetts with an office in Barnstable, on Cape Cod. I received my MD from Boston University 23 years ago in 1970, and then did a 4-year residency in pathology. I developed an interest in nutrition, preventive medicine and vitamin therapy after graduation, and proceeded to found the Cambridge Center for Holistic Health in 1976 and more recently, the Center for Preventive Medicine, in Barnstable, Massachusetts, on Cape Cod.

I am a charter member of the American Holistic Medical Association. I am a Fellow and member of the Board of Directors of the American College for Advancement in Medicine, and the Chairman of their Scientific Advisory Committee. I am a Fellow of the International Academy of Nutrition and Preventive Medicine. I have a weekly Boston area call-in radio show reporting the latest in nutrition and preventive medicine. I am also the Vice President of the American Preventive Medical Association.

I want to thank Senator Kennedy and the members of this committee for the opportunity to clarify some of the important issues regarding dietary supplements and the FDA. I am particularly eager to relay the concerns of many of my patients and radio listeners in and around Massachusetts about their continued ability to purchase all forms of dietary supplements and to have information about their use. Many ideas relating to this form of medical care and self-care are coming out of Massachusetts. You are no doubt familiar with the reports on alternative health care by Harvard physician Dr. David Eisenberg, from the recent PBS series with Bill Moyers.

One-third of all Americans are choosing to visit alternative health care practitioners and one-half take dietary supplements because they are willing to take personal responsibility for their own health. This costs the government nothing, and it can be clearly demonstrated that it will potentially save the government billions of dollars while enhancing the health of most Americans, with no significant risks.

The FDA has a long and clear history of bias against dietary supplements, recently evidenced by their attempted removal from the market of black currant oil capsules, claiming that it was an unsafe food additive and that the food to which it was being added was the gelatin capsule in which it was packaged. This was thrown out of court by three judges who said that the FDA was using "Alice-in-Wonderland reasoning in an effort to make an end-run around the law." FDA's own scientists and toxicologists testified that they were unaware of any safety problems with this oil. Following FDA's lead, the Texas Department of Health removed coenzyme Q10 from health food stores. Coenzyme Q10 is a remarkable, harmless substance that helps so many patients that I could hardly practice conscientiously without it. I have no doubt that it would be unavailable without passage of S. 784.

The FDA has disregarded or rejected competent scientific evidence that *Serenoa repens*, a standardized extract of the saw palmetto berry, can help shrink an enlarged prostate in middle-aged men. Meanwhile, another more expensive, more toxic, and less effective drug, for the same purpose, has been approved by the FDA. They knew that the published evidence showed the superiority of the *Serenoa*, but their action exposed 10 million men to unnecessary risks.

CSPI [Center for Science in the Public Interest] has referred to this bill as the "snake-oil promotion act." This is offensive to me and thousands of my colleagues who have clinically used supplements safely and effectively for many years. In fact, I started using them because of the vast medical literature substantiating their benefits. I have seen these benefits in 17 years of clinical practice. I have seen almost no side effects from these products in all these years

181

and no serious side effects. FDA-approved prescription drugs, *when used as directed*, continue to kill and injure many people annually. Dietary supplements are remarkably safe. I have been taking large amounts of them myself for many years. FDA's stated concerns about the safety of such products is not justified. Supplements are probably safer than the water that you drink to take them.

The case of L-tryptophan is important, because the FDA continues to use it as an example. It was published in both the *New England Journal of Medicine* and in the *Journal of the AMA*, in 1990, that the eosinophilia myalgia syndrome was due to a contaminant in a particular company's product. In fact, L-tryptophan has *not* been removed from the market, but only from the health food stores. It is still used in *intravenous feeding* and in *infant formulas*. The FDA has adequate safety data to permit it as an ingredient in these products.

No one wants to be the victim of fraud, and labels must be accurate. S. 784 vigorously addresses fraudulent labeling. However, *misleading labels are not as serious or dangerous a problem as the potential loss of health-enhancing dietary supplements*. But FDA's proposed regulations, which essentially ban all health claims for dietary supplements, violate the intent of the NLEA [Nutrition Labeling and Education Act]. A textbook about supplements, or scientific studies, cannot be provided by a health food store, according to FDA. Last year the *New York Times* published an article supportive of the value of dietary supplements, but a manufacturer cannot send that article, nor any supportive scientific article, to its customers without concern for potential FDA regulatory action.

FDA's spokesmen mislead by carefully selecting their words when testifying before Congress in order to avoid saying what they really intend, as evidenced by their position papers. They say the debate is not about vitamins and minerals when sold in what they call reasonable potencies. What they call reasonable is far too low to be used as a guideline for optimum health. FDA considers as a drug any higher potencies of vitamins or minerals, or dietary supplements that have no essential requirement in human nutrition, or products consumed for health enhancement or therapy. *Again, the real public health danger is from restricting access to dietary supplements, not their potential side effects.*

Specific Points

1. Without the passage of S. 784, the FDA will increase its inappropriate enforcement of misinterpreted regulations to remove a number of safe and beneficial dietary supplements from the marketplace, thus decreasing the available health choices of Americans and raising health care costs.

2. The Dietary Supplement Health and Education Act would allow these products to remain on the market with *substantiated* health claims based on scientific data. FDA and CSPI do not speak for or protect the public on this issue, and their comments are usually unsubstantiated opinion.

3. I couldn't practice medicine responsibly without many of the substances that the FDA has already tried and will continue to try to remove from the market. I base this on what I have read from their own position papers.

4. The vast majority of the population do not want the FDA to restrict dietary supplements. To call this bill simply an industry attempt to avoid regulation belittles the enormous grass roots movement in its

favor and the intelligence of the many constituents who take and depend on dietary supplements for their continued good health.

5. The FDA blatantly misrepresents the dangers of supplements when it reports to Congress that there have been deaths from vitamin A or toxicity from essential oils, which is contrary to fact.

6. It would be ridiculous in America to have restrictions on dietary supplements but ready access to alcohol, tobacco, and "Big Macs," with all their known problems.

If I could spend a half-hour with each of you, I am convinced that you would want to take at least two or three dietary supplements that the FDA has either already tried to restrict, or will without passage of S. 784. *Serenoa* for the prostate and coenzyme Q10 for the heart are good examples.

In my medical practice in Massachusetts over the past 17 years, I have seen over 10,000 patients. It is clear that many people are willing and competent to make their own choices regarding health care, including dietary supplements. They are not being duped, but they know what is at stake, and they are willing to spend their own money, not federal or state money, for the right to improve their health and prevent disease. They will not be able to continue to do this without the passage of this bill, which I strongly support.

Some of my colleagues and various researchers have also expressed similar sentiments, and I would like to report some of these to you. For example, Gladys Block, PhD, has made the following points:

1. The evidence of a beneficial role for [antioxidant] nutrients is extraordinarily extensive.

2. Many Americans are not consuming even minimal, let alone excessive, amounts of nutrients.
3. There is no evidence that supplement users neglect their diet or other health care—quite the contrary.
4. The evidence of benefit is increasing explosively, and conclusions formed a decade ago are insufficient to inform us.
5. FDA's role in protecting public health would be much more valuable if focused on ensuring quality of supplements and providing consumers with information.

In the reviews of the *Serenoa repens* extract studies published by the FDA in *New Developments*, of March 5, 1990, they gave their reasoning for not allowing claims for prostate improvement. Although they admitted that there was "statistically significant" improvement, they considered it not to be "clinically significant," even though it was better in all parameters than the drug that they did approve. The drug is potentially dangerous, and women who may get pregnant who are partners of men taking the drug are cautioned to avoid exposure to this partner's semen and to avoid handling the crushed tablets of the drug. It also has other side effects (impotence, decreased libido, ejaculation dysfunction). There are no known side effects from the herbal product.

The FDA does not consider only the value and safety of dietary supplements in deciding what to approve. It has other motives, including *"...what steps are necessary to ensure that the existence of dietary supplements on the market does not act as a disincentive for drug development."* Also, Deputy Commissioner for Policy David Adams said that the establishment of a separate regulatory category for supplements *"...could undercut the exclusivity rights enjoyed by the holders of approved drug applications."*

In a letter to the *New York Times*, September 8, 1992, Dr. Bernard Rimland said "...Dr. Kessler tells us that the FDA doesn't want to block the sale of vitamins. All we have to do is convince him and his fellow bureaucrats that they have been wrong for many decades in saying that vitamins are useless. Just provide the FDA with the evidence that will make them change their minds and they will let us buy all the vitamins we want. Fat chance! The FDA's stonewalling of any and all evidence favoring the use of vitamins is legendary. We could more easily convince a shark to become a vegetarian."

The evidence does not support the FDA claims that nutrients, including amino acids, are in any way a significant risk. These baseless claims mislead Congress and the public and make it dangerous to give such regulatory power to the FDA.

In case there is doubt about the regulatory intentions of the FDA, let me include some quotes from FDA officials pinpointing their position:

From the *Task Force Report on Dietary Supplements*:

"...the task force recommends that the agency adopt a 'Dietary Supplement Limit' which would be the maximum daily intake of a given vitamin or mineral that the agency deems safe" — e.g., "the highest RDA levels listed by the National Academy of Sciences." "The Agency should take regulatory action against those supplements that exceed the above guidelines as 'unsafe food additives'...."

"Amino acids should be regulated as drugs."

"If a potency is listed on the label for any non-essential substance (a dietary supplement for which there is no RDA) action would be taken against those products."

One has to question the rationale behind the FDA's proposal to redefine amino acids as "drugs." Using such an approach should suggest that sugar (sucrose) refined from beets or sugar cane, a food extraction product, should be regulated as a "drug." In fact, sugar in the American diet poses far more risks than amino acids.

Follow-up Testimony

Here is the text of what I wrote to the committee after the hearings were over, for inclusion in the official Congressional record of the hearings:

During the testimony at this hearing of Dr. David Kessler, Commissioner of the Food and Drug Administration, he made a number of misleading and false statements and a number of confusing points. I addressed some of those points in my testimony, but due to a lack of time I did not address all of them, nor did I respond adequately to reflect my concerns.

First of all on the issue of the safety of nutrients. The FDA has asked that dietary supplements meet the same standards of safety as OTC [over-the-counter] drugs. Using their own data and according to all the records of the American Association of Poison Control Centers, dietary supplements are 2550 times safer than OTC drugs.

Dr. Kessler said that there was potential toxicity from chromium, folic acid, gamma-linolenic acid (GLA) and L-tryptophan. I am sure that he feels there is a problem with other nutrients in spite of their long record of safety based on animal and human studies and traditional use. If Dr. Kessler *feels* there is a risk, he can avoid taking these products, but only if he can *reasonably prove* a risk should the FDA be allowed to remove these from the market.

I would like to state categorically that there is no known risk from the ingestion of any of the above products at *anywhere near* the amounts that are typically used. In fact, you would probably have to take enough GLA-containing oil to get obese from the calories before it would do any other harm. No one is recommending such high doses.

Folic acid does not cause any side effects. What Dr. Kessler calls a side effect, the masking of the anemia that is an early sign of a B12 deficiency, is actually a therapeutic benefit. However, I recognize that a B12 deficiency, if prolonged, may lead to peripheral neuropathy, but this is not a side effect of the folic acid. There are now easy ways to measure B12 in the blood, so a physician would not have any difficulty in recognizing a deficiency. You might argue that you need to see a physician to determine this even if people are taking folic acid on their own. However, that is moot, because a person would need a physician to recognize the anemia also. Although the dispute revolves around the dose of 400 to 1000 *micro*grams (mcg), folic acid is safe at doses measured in *milli*grams (mg). I have seen no side effects in patients taking up to 100 mg (100,000 mcg). This dose has been used to treat gout, because, as a xanthine oxidase inhibitor, folate works like the drug allopurinol. Inhibition of xanthine oxidase may also reduce the risk of heart disease.

Chromium is a perfectly safe nutrient that can lower cholesterol and help to regulate insulin, thus improving sugar control in diabetics and hypoglycemics. Doses that I have recommended, again with no clinical or laboratory signs of toxicity, range up to 1000 micrograms. It is safer than the drugs that are approved to lower cholesterol (e.g., lovastatin), and they have side effects such that their effect on mortality is neutral or negative.

Lovastatin actually inhibits the production of another substance, coenzyme Q10, which is very important for a healthy heart, immune function and energy production. Since coenzyme Q10 protects against heart disease, there is theoretical evidence, and also clinical studies, showing that this is a risk of taking the drug. And, as an aside, coenzyme Q10 is a substance that the Texas Department of Health, following FDA's lead, tried to remove from the health food stores in Texas.

The case of L-tryptophan deserves more comment. Dr. Kessler repeated in his testimony the claim that "they" were not sure that the eosinophilia myalgia syndrome (EMS) was due only to a contaminant. As I stated in my testimony, the *New England Journal of Medicine* and the *Journal of the AMA* both concluded that it was from a contaminant back in 1990. In the past month there have been two reports, one from the CDC by Robert Hill published in the *Journal of Contaminants and Environmental Toxicology* and one from Dr. Cluew, a professor at George Washington University, reported at a rheumatology meeting. They both concluded that the EMS was the result of a contaminant and not L-tryptophan itself.

If the FDA and Dr. Kessler do not know the older literature on the subject and they do not know the more recent literature on the subject, they are the wrong agency or the wrong personnel to be involved with the enforcement of dietary supplement regulations. There are many other reasons that I have come to this conclusion. Either we change the agency, change the personnel or specifically limit their power with strict Congressional guidelines such as mandated in S. 784.

Dr. Kessler also revealed his true intentions inadvertently when he stated that FDA was within the law to regulate dietary supplement products that were mixtures as food additives. There is no scientific rationale for removing two safe products from the market if they happen to be mixed together, just because you have the legal authority to do so.

Some products are better when they are mixed, such as GLA and vitamin E. The product lasts longer on the shelf without oxidizing because of the presence of the vitamin E. Sometimes mixtures are cheaper and sometimes they are more effective. The FDA attitude is to blow up Mount McKinley because it's there! There is no reason to expect that the FDA, with its current personnel make-up and level of authority, will suddenly start to treat dietary supplements more equitably than they have for decades.

Dr. Kessler left the impression that all the bottles of products that he displayed, in his grandstanding gesture, were labeled with false claims. He presented only one that had a false claim on the label. (No one at the hearing actually examined the label, but I have no doubt that there are occasional false claims, which generally are not a great risk to the public health.) Most of those products were properly labeled, but FDA agents were able to cajole someone at a health food store to suggest to them that the product would be useful for a specific health problem. The manufacturers or distributors are inapppropriately being held liable for the actions of retail clerks. If a clerk in a market said to take prunes for constipation, that would be an unsubstantiated health claim according to the FDA, and they could have put a box of prunes on the table with all those bottles.

When confronted with the toxicity of FDA-approved drugs, which kill so many people annually, Dr. Kessler replied with his "canned" comment that "half of our drugs are derived from plants." This is a clear misrepresentation and designed to mislead. Many pharmaceuticals are plant extracts that have been significantly altered so that they can be patented, and this alteration usually increases their toxicity. Also, many of them are synthetic analogs of plant products, not the plants themselves. You might as well say that they are made from carbon, nitrogen and oxygen, which we encounter every day! Further, many of the most widely used and most expensive drugs are totally synthetic and have nothing to do with plants. Anti-ulcer drugs, anti-inflammatory drugs, anti-anxiety drugs, newer cardiac drugs and antihypertensives are not plant products. They cost many Americans lots of money and have numerous side effects. They are necessary for many patients but are widely overused. This is partly because physicians have no access, in the normal course of their work, to the information about dietary supplements that should be disseminated widely. This would lessen the need for drugs and enhance the health of all Americans, while reducing the medical care crisis that we are now facing.

Dr. Kessler decried the variety of health claims being made for evening primrose oil. He is perhaps unaware of the hundreds of studies in the literature supporting most of those uses. It is not surprising that a physician would be skeptical of something that seems to help so many illnesses. But it is a mistake to be blinded by skepticism from seeing the scientific evidence. Because GLA [from evening primrose and other oils] is a precursor to regulatory substances known as "prostaglandins," it has wide-ranging metabolic effects. It does help to lower blood pressure, reduce or cure atopic dermatitis, relieve PMS, reduce cholesterol and inflammation and help asthmatics and allergic patients. These are the many effects of the prostaglandins that are made from this important fatty acid. It is therefore not "incredible" to someone who bothers to look up the scientific documentation and who understands the metabolic rationale.

I want to reaffirm that these claims were *not* on the labels of these products, but they *are* in the medical literature. Also, I have observed in my practice the above-stated clinical effects, and have reviewed many of the studies substantiating some of the claims that the FDA agents heard

191

from health food store clerks. The FDA should be doing everything in its power to disseminate this information and encouraging manufacturers to disseminate it also, as long as it is in the medical literature and not misleading. Instead, they are an obstacle to information exchange and are themselves misleading. This can only be changed if the FDA stops confusing its role of regulating real danger and fraud with the role of being the arbiter and promoter of truth as they see it. Passage of S. 784 will ensure a more sane approach to regulation, availability of dietary supplements and truthful health claims.

When Dr. Kessler says that they "plan to take no products off the market," that is a dramatic shift from what they have proposed in all their written material until now. With such waffling, confusion and misleading testimony, the FDA cannot be expected to take an honest and human approach to regulating such an important component of our health care.

I have read Dr. Linus Pauling's letter addressed to the committee supporting the Dietary Supplements Act. I hope it is included in the record because it is an eloquent statement that combines common sense, science, reason and compassion.

Linus Pauling's Testimony

Linus Pauling, the only person ever to have won two unshared Nobel prizes, died in 1994 at the age of 93. He pursued his research and directed the Linus Pauling Institute of Science and Medicine until shortly before his death from prostate cancer. He partially credited his long life (his parents had both died quite young) to his large doses of vitamin C (18 g per day) and other dietary supplements.

Here is the text of Linus Pauling's letter to the Senate committee, reprinted with permission of his family:

I am deeply concerned with the current state of affairs revolving around the issue of dietary supplements and related substances. The overwhelming body of evidence in the official medical and scientific indices regarding the efficacy and safety of vitamins, minerals, enzymes, amino acids, herbs, and other nutritionally related substances is obviously being ignored or, at best, misinterpreted to suit the special interests of a medical and political contingency. The volumes of respected historical data and conclusive current research in regard to these substances and their value in healthcare far outweigh single isolated instances of contamination, not to mention clinically and statistically unsubstantiated claims of toxicity. The manipulation of empirical credibility by political or economic egos is not to be tolerated or exonerated.

As a scientist, chemist, physicist, crystallographer, molecular biologist, and medical researcher, I have spent a lifetime in pursuit of expert knowledge. This issue involving the definition, regulation, and censorship of dietary supplements and associated information goes far beyond this hearing. It touches upon the very fiber of our human and constitutional rights. It mandates monopolization of the healthcare industry by creating an economic premise that will eventually eliminate those unable to meet its unrealistic requirements. These demands would require millions of dollars in research and excessive time constraints to prove the safety of substances already historically and statistically within considerable safety margins.

In the scientific and medical comunities, among those of reputable and significant knowledge, the votes have already been cast in favor of nontoxic therapies that are effective and affordable. This issue of agency determination of definitions and regulations overrides the individual's freedom of choice in healthcare, and inhibits free access to vitamin information that better enables a person to make an informed intelligent decision regarding services that could be of significant value in the prevention and treatment of disease, making it mandatory that they be made available only as "drugs," and under the jurisdiction therefore of the medical community. This ultimately enslaves a population to becoming chemically, psychologically, and economically dependent, rather than being actively responsible for its own well being. Billions of dollars and millions of lives are at risk of being jeopardized in this ruthless campaign to subjugate the health industry to being puppets of a legislated system of lobbying efforts.

It is imperative to maintain the highest quality of purity, safety, and performance in regard to consumer products and services. However, the subversive actions of raids at gunpoint, confiscation of patients' records and personal property, and warrantless censorship and banning of information and substances that are statistically proven to be of benefit are blatant violations of human and constitutional rights. As a scientist, I am appalled at the audacity of those challenging these rights; as a citizen, I am compelled to voice my indignation at being considered incapable of being in charge of my own health. The medical community needs to become a partner, not a dictator, in the healthcare system.

Over a quarter of a century ago, I became interested in nutrient compounds and their effects on human health. The old professors of nutrition who helped to develop the science of nutrition seemed complacent with their accomplishments and ignored the new discoveries that were being made in medicine, biochemistry, and molecular biology. They continued to teach their students the old ideas, many of them incomplete or incorrect, resulting in principles and practices that have denied the public proper access to new concepts and therapies.

Physicians themselves, though dedicated and intelligent, are virtually untrained in the area of nutritional science and metabolic therapy, other than conventional drug modalities and allopathic procedures. If there is to be a concerted effort to regulate and eliminate toxic substances, it would serve the issue far better to address the abuse of drugs and treatment procedures that are the cause of hundreds of thousands of medical catastrophies and deaths per year, which could possibly be avoided by improving medical education of the physicians and the public as to nutritional alternatives in healthcare maintenance.

At this hearing, I urge you to consider seriously the ramifications of crippling the full disclosure of information to the public regarding health research, and the unnecessary regulations and improper definitions of dietary supplements as drugs. This implies a direct infringemement of medical freedom of choice and the First Amendment, freedom of speech, allowing for a dangerous precedent of censorship that could generate epidemic problems not only in human health but human values. The Constitution of the World Health Organization, as mandated in conformity with the Charter of the United Nations, of which the United States is a signatory, states:

"Health is a state of complete physical, mental and social well-being and not merely the absence of disease or infirmity. The enjoyment of the highest standard of health is one of the fundamental rights of every human being without distinction of race, religion, political belief, economic or social condition. The health of all peoples is fundamental to the attainment of peace and security and is dependent upon the fullest cooperation of individuals and states. The extension to all peoples of the benefits of medical, psychological and related knowledge is essential to the fullest attainment of health. Informed opinion and active cooperation on the part of the public are of the utmost importance in the improvement of the health of the people." (Geneva, 1976)

This hearing is paramount to the determination of the Dietary Supplements Act, S-784. I submit to you the history-making moment that we are facing. As representatives of the people, consider not only the medical and scientific implications, but the humanity of your decisions. We are on the threshold of a new paradigm. The future of our self-determination as humankind depends upon our right to life and to live in freedom. Herophiles in 300 BC stated: "When Health is absent, Wisdom cannot reveal itself, Art cannot become manifest, Strength cannot be exerted, Wealth is useless, and Reason is powerless."

I trust that your reason will surpass the rhetoric, and that your wisdom will reveal the truth in support of the Dietary Supplements Act.

Sincerely,
Linus Pauling

Unfortunately, in spite of the ultimate passage of a watered down version of the Dietary Supplement Health and Education Act, there are still political, behind-the-scenes maneuverings that make it unclear what will happen with regulation and oversight of dietary supplements by the FDA. The FDA officials and lawyers have been working tirelessly to "interpret" the language of the bill to try to maintain their inappropriate restriction on availability of supplements and on access to information about them.

If you want to help ensure the continued availability of dietary supplements and your access to information about them, you can contact your representatives in Washington and let them know you want their support for this. You can also support several organizations that, as of 1995, are working toward passage of a revision of the dietary supplement bill. This will surely still be an issue for the next few years.

One of these organizations is the American Preventive Medical Association (see Appendix 2, "Resources"), which is working toward more health freedom in many ways.

Health Endangered In Canada

North of the border, dietary supplement consumers face similar problems to those in the US. And their regulations may be even worse. In 1995, the Canadian parliament has been considering a bill (C-7) which would make it difficult to find any over-the-counter dietary supplements. Because they have an effect on states of health, it is being proposed that access to supplements and information about them be restricted.

The Bill C-7 would technically criminalize anyone who sold any herbal remedy or natural supplement with stimulant or relaxant properties. Tryptophan is already a prescription drug in Canada, and its price has risen dramatically since losing its over-the-counter status. (At least it is available, unlike in the US.)

Other substances that are harmful to health are being specifically exempted from coverage by this bill. Thus, Canadians may be in the ridiculous position of being able to buy nicotine, alcohol and caffeine freely but not large doses of vitamin C or vitamin E. It can hardly be argued that the main goal of this bill is to protect public health. There is also an exemption for prescription drugs, which are at least 2500 times more dangerous than dietary supplements. There are Canadian associations that are working against this bill. (See Appendix 2, "Resources.")

Chapter 14

Conclusion

This has been a brief overview of the use of nutrient supplements in health care and health-oriented medicine. It gives you a good foundation for establishing your own supplement regimen as part of your total health program. If you have serious health problems you would be wise to seek the advice of a health professional—and wisest to look for one who is nutritionally oriented. Working together you can plan a total health program for your individual needs.

As you can see, most dietary supplements that are specific nutrients are useful for both prevention and treatment, while the herbal supplements are more frequently valuable for treatment of specific health problems. There are some exceptions, for example, echinacea and silymarin, which are helpful for immune enhancement and liver protection if you take them periodically while you are healthy. Many herbal products are also helpful in minor acute illnesses or as first aid treatments.

Try Supplements First

It is clear that *many conditions that are treated with drugs should be treated first with a proper total health program and dietary supplements.* If the situation is an emergency, then I am all in favor of immediate and appropriate medical or surgical treatments. However, even in these circumstances, nutrients might be the first choice. Recent studies have shown that magnesium infusions for heart attack patients can significantly reduce serious complications and deaths. It can also be a first line of treatment for acute asthma. If health problems do not respond to nutrition, dietary supplements, exercise and stress reduction, medicine and surgery are still available.

Most health problems are not emergencies. To treat them as though they were chronic, recurrent emergencies, which is the way medicine is often practiced today, is costly, time consuming and generally ineffective. It causes many problems, often more than it relieves, and these are sometimes deadly. Side effects of medications kill more people annually than automobile accidents. Unnecessary surgery (heart disease and other conditions) has significant mortality while it also drives up health care costs. This approach to health care also takes the power and responsibility for your health out of your control.

Your Personal Power for Health

The intensity of debate in government circles that revolves around solving the "health care crisis" is misguided, misinformed, and misnamed. It has nothing to do with health, but is really an effort to find ways to pay for the excess disease care that too many Americans need. They need this extra care because they do not take proper care of their personal health. You can personally do more than the entire government toward solving the health crisis and the cost of medical care—simply by taking care of yourself and decreasing your own costs of health care.

While the government can do little to solve the larger health crisis, there is much that you can do for yourself that will have a far greater impact on your own health than any government program. It is a mistake to think that the government is honestly interested in health when they allow fast food companies to provide the food services at schools, and when high government officials set the wrong example by having "photo-ops"of themselves in the local "burger-fries-and-a-shake" joint, even if they jog to get there.

You do not have to accept this situation. Ultimately, you are responsible for your own health. I once saw a mock ad in a health magazine that said, "Wanted: Reformers; not of the government but of themselves." It must begin with you.

If you are ill or just not feeling up to par, you should know that *in most circumstances you have the power to create your own health.* You can do it with simple lifestyle changes and dietary supplements. If you need education and professional advice to begin your path to self-determined health, you have already started by reading this book.

Appendix 1

Dietary Allowances

Recommended Dietary Allowances

The Recommended Dietary Allowances (RDA) are designed to prevent deficiency diseases in most healthy people. But deficiency diseases such as scurvy and beriberi are not the problems of the civilized world. These are the RDAs, as set forth by the Food and Nutrition Board of the National Research Council.

Vitamin A (& beta-carotene)* .... 5000/4000 IU
Vitamin C .... 60 mg
Vitamin D .... 200 IU
Vitamin E* .... 15/12 IU
Vitamin K* .... 80/60 mcg
Thiamin (B1)* .... 1.5/1.1 mg
Riboflavin (B2)* .... 1.7/1.3 mg
Niacin (& niacinamide; B3)* .... 19/15 mg
Pyridoxine (B6)* .... 2.0/1.6 mg
Folate (folic acid)* .... 0.2/0.18 mg
Cobalamin (B12) .... 2 mcg
Biotin* .... 0.3 mg
Pantothenic acid (B5)* .... 4/7 mg
Calcium .... 800 mg

Iron* .... 10/15 mg
Phosphorus ....800 mg
Iodine .... 150 mcg
Magnesium* ....350/280 mg
Zinc ....15 mg
Copper .... 1.5–3 mg
Sodium .... 500 mg
Potassium .... 2000 mg
Selenium* .... 70/55 mcg

*Second value is for women.

Daily Values

On food and supplement labels, you will see nutrients listed as "Percent Daily Value," or the relative amount of that nutrient in a portion of food, compared to another standard of dietary needs. This "DV" amount is different from the RDA.

Vitamin A (& beta-carotene) .... 5000 IU
Vitamin C.. 60 mg
Vitamin D.. 400 IU
Vitamin E .... 30 IU
Thiamin (B1)... 1.5 mg
Riboflavin (B2).. 1.7 mg
Niacin (& niacinamide; B3) .... 20 mg
Pyridoxine (B6)... 2.0 mg
Folate (folic acid) .... 0.4 mg
Cobalamin (B12) .... 6.0 mcg
Biotin .... 0.3 mg

Pantothenic acid (B5) .... 10 mg
Calcium .... 1000 mg
Iron .... 18 mg
Phosphorus .... 1000 mg
Iodine .... 150 mcg
Magnesium .... 400 mcg
Zinc .... 15 mg
Copper .... 2 mg
Sodium .... 2500 mg
Potassium .... 4000 mg

There are no Daily Values for other nutrients, such as vitamin K, manganese, selenium and chromium, but this does not mean they are unimportant.

Healthy Dietary Allowances

My own recommendations of minimums for basic health are clearly different from the RDA levels and the Daily Values. They reflect both food sources and extra nutrients derived from dietary supplements.

For basic preventive medicine, free-radical protection, and health enhancement I recommend:

Vitamin A (& beta-carotene) .... 25,000 IU
Vitamin C .... 4,000 mg
Vitamin D .... 400 IU
Vitamin E .... 400 IU
Thiamin (B1) .... 100 mg
Riboflavin (B2) .... 50 mg
Niacin (& niacinamide; B3) .... 150 mg
Pyridoxine (B6) .... 100 mg

Folate (folic acid) .... 5,000 mcg
Cobalamin (B12) .... 100 mcg
Biotin .... 0.3 mg
Pantothenic acid (B5) .... 100 mg
Calcium .... 500 mg
Iron .... 18 mg
Phosphorus .... 1,000 mg
Iodine .... 150 mcg
Magnesium .... 500 mg
Zinc .... 30 mg
Copper .... 3 mg
Sodium .... 1,000 mg
Potassium .... 4,000 mg

Notice that my recommended level for sodium is *lower* than the DV. It is more a reflection of need than the DV, since excess sodium is unhealthy. The DV is based, in part, on what people are actually getting from food, rather than what is ideal for health. Since consumption of salt is usually so high (5000–13,000 mg daily!), the DV is actually above what you really need.

My recommendation for calcium is also lower than the RDA. This is predicated on your eating a healthier diet than the one common in the United States and many other industrialized countries. If you eat too much protein (especially animal protein), caffeine, sugar, salt, and sodas, then you will very likely need more calcium. You may also need more calcium if you lead a sedentary lifestyle, although more dietary calcium is no substitute for weight-bearing exercise, such as walking or jogging, if maintaining bone density is one of your goals. If you have adequate magnesium nutrition, it is probably quite safe to take extra calcium.

Older standards suggested getting twice as much calcium as magnesium. This was based on the ratio of the two minerals in the blood, and does not necessarily reflect dietary needs. Variations in absorption, utilization, and the physiology of the two minerals make the blood levels unreliable figures for determining dietary needs.

Magnesium deficiencies are quite common, marginal deficiencies are difficult to detect, and long-term consequences of low magnesium intake are quite serious. They include neurologic, heart and kidney diseases. For these reasons I recommend at least as much magnesium as calcium. High calcium intake also increases the need for magnesium.

A healthy diet naturally contains a lot of potassium. However, people taking certain diuretics or those eating a large amount of salt may need potassium supplements.

Appendix 2

Resources

If you need further advice from a health- or nutrition-oriented professional, there is a growing body of physicians who can help you. The number of medical doctors interested in this field is increasing rapidly. The membership in the American College for Advancement in Medicine, for example, has doubled to more than 725 in the past few years, and most of the members are experienced in dietary supplements. There is also an American Holistic Medical Association, and the American Academy of Environmental Medicine, whose members also often have some interest in this field. In addition there are many naturopathic physicians (ND) and certified nutritionists (CN) who may be able to help you.

Not surprisingly, many health food store managers have a lot of information on the value of dietary supplements. Unfortunately, because of the legal-political situation, they have to be very circumspect in what information they give out. Sometimes they are only willing to recommend books or articles because even any accurate information they give out is considered mislabeling by the FDA. As the political situation is changing, you may find increasing information available through many sources.

There is also much further reading that you can do, whether you are educating yourself for your own health or you are a professional looking to help your patients. There are many books written by experienced professionals giving practical guidelines and background information. This Appendix is only a partial listing of the books that I recommend. Each one will give many other sources if you wish to pursue more intense study. Some of the books are older and may be out of print, but they will usually be available in the library. They contain valuable background information and further references.

No one book has all the answers, and often the books will disagree with each other on some points, but in general there is wide agreement about the value of different dietary supplements. Whatever you read, make sure you apply some of your own common sense to the material before accepting it. If you see health practitioners for guidance, whether medical doctors, naturopaths, acupuncturists, chiropractors, nutritionists, or others, be sure to ask questions in order to be fully informed about your treatment.

General Books

Steve Austin, ND, and Cathy Hitchcock, MSW
  Breast Cancer: What You Should Know (But May Not Be Told) About Prevention, Diagnosis, and Treatment

James Balch, MD, and Phyllis Balch, CN
  Prescription for Nutritional Healing

Jeffrey Bland, PhD
  Your Health Under Siege, Using Nutrition to Fight Back

Arline Brecher
  Forty-Something Forever

James P. Carter, MD, DrPH
  Racketeering in Medicine: The Suppression of Alternatives

Emmanuel Cheraskin, MD, DMD

The Vitamin C Connection
Diet and Disease
Psychodietetics
New Hope for Incurable Diseases
Predictive Medicine
Vitamin C: Who Needs It?

Norman Cousins

Anatomy of an Illness
The Healing Heart
Head First

Elmer Cranton, MD

Bypassing Bypass: The New Technique of Chelation Therapy

William G. Crook, MD

The Yeast Connection

Udo Erasmus

Fats That Heal, Fats That Kill

Alan Gaby, MD

B6, The Natural Healer
Preventing and Reversing Osteoporosis

Abram Hoffer, MD, PhD

Nutrients to Age Without Senility
Orthomolecular Nutrition

Beatrice Trum Hunter

Consumer Beware! Your Food and What's Been
Done to It
The Mirage of Safety: Food Additives and Federal Policy
The Great Nutrition Robbery
Food Additives and Your Health

Richard Kunin, MD
  Mega-Nutrition

Michael Murray, ND, and Joseph Pizzorno, ND
  A Textbook of Natural Medicine
  Encyclopedia of Natural Medicine

Richard Passwater, PhD
  Supernutrition
  Supernutrition for a Healthy Heart

Linus Pauling, PhD
  Vitamin C and the Common Cold
  Vitamin C, the Common Cold, and the Flu
  Cancer and Vitamin C
  How to Live Longer and Feel Better

Patrick Quillin, PhD, RD
  Healing Nutrients
  Beating Cancer with Nutrition

John Robbins
  Diet for a New America

Bill Gottlieb, Editor
  New Choices in Natural Healing

Donald Rudin, MD, and Clara Felix
  The Omega-3 Phenomenon

Judy Shabert, MD, RD, and Nancy Ehrlich
  The Ultimate Nutrient: Glutamine

Charles B. Simone, MD
  Cancer and Nutrition

Irwin Stone
  The Healing Factor: Vitamin C Against Disease

Martin J. Walker

Dirty Medicine: Science, big business and the assault on natural health care

Julian Whitaker, MD

Reversing Heart Disease
Reversing Diabetes
Reversing Health Risks
Is Heart Surgery Necessary?

Jonathan Wright, MD

Dr. Wright's Book of Nutritional Therapy
Dr. Wright's Guide to Healing with Nutrition

Periodicals/Newsletters

Natural Health

Vegetarian Times

Vegetarian Journal
Vegetarian Resource Group

Longevity

Health and Healing Newsletter
Julian Whitaker, MD, editor; Phillips Publishing, telephone: 800-777-5005 or 301-424-3700

Nutrition and Healing Newsletter
Jonathan Wright, MD, with Alan Gaby, MD; telephone: 800-528-0559

Health Notes
Skye Lininger, DC, editor; at health food stores

Your Health
Newsletter of the International Academy of Nutrition and Preventive Medicine, PO Box 18433, Asheville, NC 28814

Nutrition News
> Siri Khalsa; at health food stores

Health Line
> Newsletter of the International Health Foundation, PO Box 3494, Jackson, TN 38303

Canadian Periodicals

The above magazines are available in Canada, but there are also two magazines that are published in Canada:

Alive, Canadian Journal of Health and Nutrition
> at health food stores

Health Naturally, Canada's Self-Health Care Magazine
> by subscription or through magazine and health food stores

On-Line Computer Resources

Health data can be retrieved from many computer network sources, including the Internet. The following are the easiest to access and deal directly with issues discussed in this book.

Compuserve Natural Medicine Forum (GO NATMED)
> On-line discussions of many health issues and dietary supplements. Extensive library of articles on politics, dietary supplements, nutrition, medical conditions, nutrition software programs, herbs, and other healing methods. For information on Compuserve membership call 800-848-8990. Ask for operator 525 for a free sign-up kit.

Alternative Medicine Connection (ARxC)

Bulletin board and information source on chelation therapy, health, nutrition, dietary suplements, and the current political situation. Retrieve and post messages and articles. For information call 703-471-4734, or by modem dial 703-471-8465.

Other online services such as America Online and Prodigy

Discussion groups and resources on health are available, and there are also Internet discussions on alternative medicine that can be found under several headings.

Professional Books

Jeffrey Bland, PhD, Editor

Medical Applications of Clinical Nutrition
1984–1985 Yearbook of Nutritional Medicine
1986, A Year in Nutritional Medicine

Rebecca Flynn, MS, and Mark Roest

Guide to Standardized Herbal Products

William F. Ganong, MD

Review of Medical Physiology, 15th ed.

J.B. Harborne, Editor

The Flavonoids: Advances in Research Since 1986

Frank Katch and William McArdle

Introduction to Nutrition, Exercise and Health, 4th ed.

Stephen A. Levine, PhD, and Parris Kidd, PhD

Antioxidant Adaptation: Its Role in Free Radical Pathology

Maria Linder, PhD, Editor
Nutritional Biochemistry and Metabolism

Robert K. Murray, et al.
Harper's Biochemistry, 22nd ed.

Maurice Shils, MD, ScD, et al.
Modern Nutrition in Health and Disease, 8th ed.

Gene A. Spiller, PhD
Current Topics in Nutrition and Disease, Volume 4: Nutritional Pharmacology

Melvin Werbach, MD
Nutritional Influences on Illness
Nutritional Influences on Mental Illness

Melvin Werbach, MD, and Michael Murray, ND
Botanical Influences on Illness

Professional Journals and Reviews

Journal of Advancement in Medicine
Original and review articles on advances in medical care, chelation therapy, and nutrition. American College for Advancement in Medicine; for subscription telephone: 800-532-3688 or 714-583-7666.

CP Currents
Journal abstracts of worldwide literature on nutrition and preventive medicine. ITServices, For subscription, telephone: 916-483-1085.

Clinical Pearls News
Health letter on current research. Includes many relevant articles from the collection in *CP Currents*

plus interviews with researchers on timely topics in nutrition, health care and dietary supplements. ITServices.

International Clinical Nutrition Reviews
Review articles and abstracts of the world literature on nutrition and dietary suppements. Integrated Therapies, PTY Ltd, PO Box 370, Manly 2095, NSW, Australia.

Journal of Orthomolecular Medicine
Canadian Schizophrenia Foundation, 16 Florence Avenue, Toronto, Ont, M2N 1E9; telephone: 416-733-2117. They also have available many professional article reprints on nutrition and vitamin therapy.

Journal of Applied Nutrition
Original reports, reviews and commentary. International Academy of Nutrition and Preventive Medicine, PO Box 18433, Asheville, NC 28814; telephone: 704-258-3243.

Journal of Optimal Nutrition

Journal of Nutrition & Environmental Medicine (UK)
Carfax Publishing Company, PO Box 25, Abingdon, Oxfordshire, OX14 3UE, UK.

Planta Medica

Alternative and Complementary Therapies

American Journal of Clinical Nutrition

Nutrition Reviews

Journal of Naturopathic Medicine

Protocol Journal of Botanical Medicine

Professional Conference Tapes

Conferences of most of the medical organizations that teach nutrition and innovative medical treatments are recorded for later review or for those who were unable to attend the meetings. They are a good source of further education for professionals and interested lay people. They may also have a catalogue of other lectures.

Audio tapes of the American College for Advancement in Medicine (ACAM) conferences from 1994 on are available from Professional Audio Recording, telephone: 800-430-4727 or 909-593-1862; call for their catalogue of other conference tapes.

Audio tapes of ACAM conferences prior to November 1994 are available from InstaTape; telephone: 800-669-8273 or 818-303-2531. Call for their catalogue.

Audio tapes of the American Academy of Environmental Medicine conferences are available from InstaTape; telephone: 800-303-2531 or 818-303-2531.

Organizations

There are a number of organizations of health professionals that can help you locate a practitioner in your area. Starting with any of these, you should be able to find medical and nutritional support for your health needs if you have persistent problems. You may wish to start a program with a professional to help you. Some of the organizations also have members from Canada, and ACAM has many foreign members, including Canadian physicians. There are also several lay organizations doing political work and public education both in the US and in Canada. This is a list of the most active organizations.

American College for Advancement in Medicine (ACAM)

23121 Verdugo Dr., Suite 204, Laguna Hills, CA 92653; telephone toll free: 800-532-3688 or 714-583-7666; FAX: 714-455-9679. Internet domain address: www.acam.org.

For the past 20 years ACAM has been providing physician training and scientific conferences on the latest findings and emerging procedures in preventive/ nutritional medicine, as well as chelation therapy for vascular disease and other degenerative disorders. ACAM's goals are to improve physician skills, knowledge and diagnostic procedures and to develop public awareness of alternative methods of medical treatment. They publish a quarterly medical journal, the *Journal of Advancement in Medicine.*

ACAM scientific conferences and physician trainings are held twice each year in different locations around the US. The scientific conferences are open to the public as well as professionals.

American Preventive Medical Association (APMA)

459 Walker Rd., Great Falls, VA 22066; telephone toll free: 800-230-2762 or 703-759-0662; FAX: 703-759-6711

The APMA was formed as a response to the actions of the FDA and state medical licensing boards against physicians practicing nutrition and other innovative medical treatments. It is a political action group of physicians and the public. Their mission is to achieve a health care system in which practitioners can practice in good conscience, with the well-being of the patient foremost in their minds, and without fear of recrimination. They are constantly monitoring and taking an active role in the drafting of legislation.

American Holistic Medical Association (AHMA)

4101 Lake Boone Trail, Suite 201, Raleigh, NC 27607; telephone: 919-787-5181; FAX: 919-787-4916

The AHMA was founded in 1978 to unite fully licensed physicians who practice holistic medicine. Their mission is to support practitioners in their evolving personal and professional development and to promote an art and science which acknowledges all aspects of the individual, the family and the planet. Holistic medicine encompasses all safe modalities of diagnosis and treatment while emphasizing the whole person.

American Academy of Environmental Medicine (AAEM)

4510 W. 89th St., Prairie Village, KS 66207; telephone 913-642-6062; FAX: 913-341-3625

AAEM is dedicated to the purpose of education in the recognition, treatment, and prevention of illnesses induced by exposures to biologic and chemical agents encountered in air, food, and water. They have annual instructional courses in allergy and environmental medicine clinical methods and annual scientific meetings for physicians. AAEM publishes a newsletter—*The Environmental Physician* and a professional journal—*Environmental Medicine.*

American Academy for Anti-Aging Medicine (A4M)

1510 W. Montana, Chicago, IL 60614; telephone: 312-528-1000; FAX: 312-929-5733

The A4M is a medical organization that provides information on the advances in the science of longevity and anti-aging medicine. Their mission is to identify, disseminate, and promote information on biomedically valid, effective medical treatment options that retard, stabilize, or reverse the deleterious effects of the human aging process. They hold annual scientific conferences and publish the audio tapes, video tapes and proceedings.

International Academy of Nutrition and Preventive Medicine (IANPM)

PO Box 18433, Asheville, NC 28814; telephone: 704-258-3243

IANPM actively supports the use of nutrition and preventive medicine in the health care system. They publish the peer-reviewed *Journal of Applied Nutrition* and a newsletter, *Your Health*

American Association of Naturopathic Physicians

PO Box 20386, Seattle, WA 98112; telephone: 206-328-8510

Founded in 1985, the AANP is the national association representing naturopathic physicians. Naturopathic physicians are primary health care providers who use nontoxic therapies such as clinical nutrition, homeopathy, botanical medicine, hydrotherapy, physical medicine and counseling. The AANP represents approximately 500 licensed naturopathic doctors.

Cancer Treatment Research Foundation
Alta Dalton, 8181 S. Lewis, Tulsa, OK 74137; telephone: 800-795-9579; FAX: 918-496-5715

They hold regular conferences on adjuvant nutrition in the treatment and management of cancer.

Society for Orthomolecular Medicine of America (SOMA)
2698 Pacific Ave., San Francisco, CA 94115 Telephone: 415-346-2500

This is a professional association of physicians practicing nutrition and dietary supplement therapy, as well as other innovative medical treatments.

Citizens for Health (CFH)
PO Box 1195, Tacoma, WA 98401; telephone: 800-357-2211 or 206-922-2457; FAX: 206-922-7583

Citizens for Health is a grass roots political organization working toward freedom of choice in health care and public access to dietary supplements and information about them. They work on a national and state level and have chapters in all 50 United States, Canada, and other countries.

Physicians and Scientists for a Healthy World (PSHW)
171 Abbeyhill Drive, Kanata, ON K2L 2E9 or FAX: 613-831-2523

This Canadian organization is battling parliament Bill C-7, in order to protect consumers' rights and the availability of health foods, dietary supplements and information about them. They state in their petition on the bill, "Preventive health is my responsibility and therefore it must be my freedom to choose what I feel is the best wellness program for myself and my family without government interference."

My Health/My Rights (MHMR)
16 Marquis Ave., Etobicoke, Ont., M8X 1V4; Telephone: 416-233-1689 or 613-957-0200 (Québec)

MHMR is a society founded by consumers to inform and protect the rights of consumers in health related matters, including access to dietary supplements, other safe treatments, and information about them.

List of Abbreviations

A4M .... American Academy of Anti-Aging Medicine
AAEM .... American Academy of Environmental Medicine
AANP .... American Association of Naturopathic Physicians
ACAM .... American College for Advancement in Medicine
AHMA .... American Holistic Medical Association
AIDS .... Acquired immune deficiency syndrome
APMA .... American Preventive Medical Association
ARxC .... Alternative Medicine Connection
ATP .... Adenosine triphosphate
BPH .... Benign prostatic hypertrophy
CDC .... Centers for Disease Control and Prevention
CFIDS .... Chronic fatigue immune deficiency syndrome
CN .... Certified Nutritionist
CoQ10 .... Coenzyme Q10
CSPI .... Center for Science in the Public Interest
DDT .... Dichlorodiphenyl trichloroethane
DGL .... Deglycyrrhizinated licorice
DHA .... Docosahexaenoic acid
DHEA .... Dehydroepiandrosterone
DLPA .... DL-Phenylalanine
DMG .... Dimethyl glycine
DNA .... Deoxyribonucleic acid
DV .... Daily values
EFA .... Essential fatty acids
EMS .... Eosinophilia myalgia syndrome
EPA .... Eicosapentaenoic acid (also Environmental
                 Protection Agency)

FDA .... United States Food and Drug Administration
GABA .... Gamma-aminobutyric acid
GLA .... Gamma-linolenic acid
GMP .... Good Manufacturing Practices
GTF .... Glucose tolerance factor
HDL .... High-density lipoprotein
IANPM ...... International Academy of Nutrition and Preventive Medicine
LDL .... Low-density lipoprotein
LPA .... L-Phenylalanine
MD .... Doctor of Medicine
MHMR ...... My Health/My Rights
MSG .... Monosodium glutamate
ND .... Doctor of Naturopathy
NLEA .... Nutrition Labeling and Education Act
NSAIDS ..... Nonsteroidal anti-inflammatory drugs
OTC .... Over-the-counter
PABA .... Para-aminobenzoic acid
PAC .... Proanthocyanidins
PBS .... Public Broadcasting System
PGE_1 .... Prostaglandin E_1
PMS .... Premenstrual syndrome
PSHW .... Physicians and Scientists for a Healthy World
RD .... Registered Dietitian
RDA .... Recommended Dietary Allowances
RNA .... Ribonucleic acid
SOD .... Superoxide dismutase
SOMA .... Society for Orthomolecular Medicine of America
T3 .... Triiodothyronine (thyroid hormone)
T4 .... Thyroxine (thyroid hormone)
USDA .... United States Department of Agriculture

Index

Dimethyl glycine
  DMG 78
  and immune function 78
DLPA
  chronic pain 105
Dolomite
  as magnesium source 84

E

Echinacea 123
  antiviral 123
  how to take 124
  interferon 123
  T-cell activity 123
  treating infections 123
  white blood cells 123
Eczema
  essential fatty acids 94
  gamma-linolenic acid 99
Eisenberg, David 180
Environmental illness
  vitamin C 68
Environmental toxins 33
EPA 97
  eicosapentaenoic acid 97
  how to take 97
  prostaglandin E3 97
Erasmus, Udo 96
Essential fatty acids 93, 94
  cell membranes 94
  hormones 94
Essential nutrients 27
Evening primrose oil. *See*
    Gamma-linolenic acid
Exercise 25
"Expensive urine" 24

F

Fatigue
  causes 161
  and food allergens 161
  L-glutamine 103

magnesium 84
  treatment program 161
Fats and oils
  animal fats 93
  hydrogenated fats 93
  inflammation 93
  saturated fats 93
  trans fats 93
  unsaturated fats 93
  vegetable fats 93
FDA 177
  intent to regulate supplements
    189
  misleading Congress
    186, 187, 189, 190
  misrepresentations 184
Feverfew 128
  histamine inhibitor 128
  how to take 129
  serotonin production 128
Fibrocystic breast disease
  vitamin E 58
Fish oils
  arthritis 97
  DHA 97
  EPA 97
  inflammation 97
Flavonoids 28, 113
  anti-allergic effects 114
  anti-inflammatory effects 114
  antioxidants 113
  antiviral effects 114
  cancer protection 113
  cataract prevention 113
  heart disease protection 113
  mixed bioflavonoids 115
  with vitamin C 113
Flax seeds and oil 98
  fiber source 98
  how to take 98
  omega-3 oil 95, 98
  spastic colon 98
Fluoride 33

Support your local bookstore. If you can't find this book,
you can order it directly from the publisher.

Order Form

*Fully guaranteed. If you are ever dissatisfied with your
purchase for any reason you may return it for a full refund.*

Telephone orders: Call Toll Free: **(800) 398-8851**. Have your
                          Discover, VISA, MasterCard or AMEX ready.
                          Telephone: (603) 878-1561

Fax orders: (603) 878-0811

On-line orders: Arcadia Press
                          1arcadia@compuserve.com

Postal orders: Arcadia Press, 161 Merriam Hill Rd.,
                          PO Box 205, Greenville, NH 03048, USA

Please send: _____ copies, @ $12.95, of *The Vitamin Revolution in
                          Health Care* by Michael Janson, MD.
                          Physicians call for quantity prices for
                          your office and your patients.

Shipping: Book rate: $3.00 shipping for the first copy, and
                          1.00 for each additional copy. Air mail $4.00 per
                          book. Foreign orders: Inquire for shipping costs.

Ship to: **Name:** _____

          Address: _____

          City: _____ **State:** _____ **Zip:**_____

          Country:_____ **Postal code:** _____

          Telephone:_____

❑ Check (Payable to Arcadia Press)
❑ Credit card: ❑ Discover, ❑ VISA, ❑ MasterCard, ❑ AMEX

Card Number_____

Signature_____Exp.date: ____ /__

Call *toll free* and order now
1-800-398-8851
Give the gift of health. Give *The Vitamin Revolution*

Support your local bookstore. If you can't find this book,
you can order it directly from the publisher.

Order Form

***Fully guaranteed. If you are ever dissatisfied with your
purchase for any reason you may return it for a full refund.***

Telephone orders:	Call Toll Free: **(800) 398-8851**. Have your Discover, VISA, MasterCard or AMEX ready. Telephone: (603) 878-1561
Fax orders:	(603) 878-0811
On-line orders:	Arcadia Press 1arcadia@compuserve.com
Postal orders:	Arcadia Press, 161 Merriam Hill Rd., PO Box 205, Greenville, NH 03048, USA
Please send: _____	copies, @ $12.95, of *The Vitamin Revolution in Health Care* by Michael Janson, MD. **Physicians** call for quantity prices for your office and your patients.
Shipping:	Book rate: $3.00 shipping for the first copy, and 1.00 for each additional copy. Air mail $4.00 per book. Foreign orders: Inquire for shipping costs.

Ship to: **Name:** _____

Address: _____

City: _____ **State:** _____ **Zip:**_____

Country:_____ **Postal code:** _____

Telephone:_____

❑ Check (Payable to Arcadia Press)
❑ Credit card: ❑ Discover, ❑ VISA, ❑ MasterCard, ❑ AMEX

Card Number_____

Signature_____Exp.date: ___ /__

Call *toll free* and order now
<u>1-800-398-8851</u>
Give the gift of health. Give *The Vitamin Revolution*